Should I take...
PROBIOTICS?

Dr. Shaun Holt

Contents

Introduction - About the Author, Copyright Statement   1

Chapter 1 - What are probiotics?   3

Chapter 2 - Products   13

Chapter 3 - How they work   23

Chapter 4 - Gastro-intestinal diseases   29

Chapter 5 - Non Gastro-intestinal diseases   49

Chapter 6 - Safety   69

Appendix - Further reading   73

About the Author

Dr. Shaun Holt is the founder of two clinical trials organizations and Research Review, a company that produces regular reviews of the medical literature for health professionals. Shaun holds Pharmacy and Medicine degrees, has been the Principal Investigator in over 50 clinical trials and has over 160 publications in the medical literature. He is the Science Director of HoneyLab, an advisor to the Asthma and Respiratory Foundation and Natural Products New Zealand, a regular contributor on TV One's Breakfast program and national radio shows. Shaun lectures at the Victoria University of Wellington, is on the editorial board of two complementary medicine journals and has previously written six books on health topics. In 2015 he was one of three finalists for the New Zealander of the Year Awards - Sanitarium Innovator of the Year. More information can be found at http://flavors.me/shaunholt

Disclaimer

The information contained in this book is intended to provide accurate and helpful health information for the general public. It is made available with the understanding that the author and publisher are not engaged in rendering medical, health, psychological, or any other kind of personal professional services in this book. The information should not be considered complete and does not cover all diseases, ailments, physical conditions or their treatment. It should not be used in place of a call or visit to a medical, health or other competent professional, who should be consulted before adopting any of the suggestions in this site or drawing inferences from it.

The information about health products contained in this book is general in nature. It does not cover all possible uses, actions, precautions, side effects, or interactions of the products mentioned, nor is the information intended as medical advice for individual problems or for making an evaluation as to the risks and benefits of taking a particular health product.

The author and publishers specifically disclaim all responsibility for any liability, loss or risk, personal or otherwise, which is incurred as a consequence, directly or indirectly, of the use and application of any of the material in this book.

First published May, 2015, Tauranga, New Zealand

ISBN: 978-0-9876617-2-2

Text © Dr. Shaun Holt. This book is copyright. Apart from any fair dealing for the purposes of private study, research, criticism or review, as permitted under the Copyright Act, no part may be reproduced by any proves without the permission of the authors.

Chapter 1
WHAT ARE PROBIOTICS?

THE UNKNOWN ORGAN

Did you know that everyone has quite a large organ in their body that they do not even know about? Or that 90% of the total number of cells in your body are not even human?

The human body is estimated to contain more than 100 trillion bacteria at any time - that is nearly 2.5kg of these tiny single-celled organisms. The mouth alone contains several hundred species of bacteria. Our bodies contain trillions of cells, and it has been estimated that in a typical human body there are at least 10 times as many cells as there are stars in the Milky Way. However, only about one in 10 of these cells are human - the remaining 90% are microbes. It is estimated that these microbes have around a hundred times as many genes in total as there are in the human genome. Because they are so small, however, they account for only a few percent, much less than 10%, of our body weight.

The bacteria in your body, if they were all collected and put in a container, would be around the size of a human liver, the large organ in the right side of the upper abdomen. As the microbiome (all the bacteria and other microbes that live in our bodies) undertake a number of important biological and physical roles in the body, in practice, it behaves as an additional body organ. Somewhere between 300 and 1,000 different species live in our gut/bowels/digestive tract, and around 99% of these bacteria come from around 30 or 40 species.

Each of our bodies has its own unique microbiome. The reason that this is different in everyone, is that it develops over the years, from birth onwards and is affected by our unique genes, our diet, and also the microbes that we are exposed to. These microbes are from many sources including our food and drink; from other people; from animals including the family dog or cat; from our environment e.g. eating mud as a child; and more recently, how many courses of antibiotics we have taken (as these kill both harmful and beneficial bacteria). People have been described by microbiologists as sponges which pick up microbes throughout our life. We carry these microbes everywhere, but the areas with the highest concentrations are the ears, nose, mouth, vagina, skin, and as we will discuss in detail, the digestive tract.

BACTERIA - GOOD AND BAD

It is important to realize that microbes, and particularly bacteria, can be "good" or "bad". In terms of being bad, this is easy to understand. Throughout human history infections have killed hundreds of millions of people. For hundreds of years until around 200 years ago, average life expectancy was only 25 years. The reason for this was that so many children and young adults died because of infections caused by microbes, such as tuberculosis, plague, influenza, typhoid, malaria and polio, to name just a few. A small wound or even a tooth abscess could be fatal, as without good treatments, infections would rapidly grow out of control and be fatal.

Thankfully, since the discovery of antibiotics, starting with the discovery of penicillin by Alexander Fleming in 1928, and with the development of vaccines, most infections that would previously have killed millions can now easily be prevented or treated. Unfortunately, bacteria are fighting back and becoming resistant to many antibiotics. For example MRSA (Methicillin-resistant Staphylococcus aureus) is resistant to almost all antibiotics and costs health systems around the world hundreds of millions of dollars. The World Health Organization (WHO) has described antibiotic resistance as the biggest threat to human health, and in 2014 President Obama signed an Executive Order directing the establishment of the Task Force for Combating Antibiotic-Resistant Bacteria.

So it would be easy to assume that all bacteria are harmful, or at the very least potentially harmful, but this is not the case, and this is the reason for writing this book. Some microbes, particularly bacteria, can actually improve our health. More than that, we actually need a lot of bacteria in our bodies to be healthy. The Human Microbiome Project (HMP) is a United States National Institutes of Health initiative which has the goal of identifying and characterizing the micro-organisms which are found in association with both healthy and diseased humans. It was launched in 2008 with a budget of US$115 million, and part of the work involves sequencing the genes of over 3,000 different bacteria. They have stated that bacteria in the gastro-intestinal tract are essential to allow people to digest foods and absorb certain nutrients. In addition, these essential microbes produce beneficial compounds such as certain vitamins, and also produce protective anti-inflammatory compounds that humans cannot produce by themselves but need for optimal health. To give just a few examples:

- Carbohydrates that humans cannot digest without bacterial help include certain starches, fibre, oligosaccharides and sugars.
- Gut bacteria are essential for the synthesis of vitamins including biotin and folate (both B vitamins).
- They are needed for the absorption of minerals including magnesium, calcium and iron.

INTERESTING FACTS ABOUT BACTERIA

- Drying your hands with paper towels will reduce the bacterial count on your hands by around 50%. But using a hand dryer will increase the bacteria on your hands by up to 250% as it blows out bacteria already living in the dryer, which has a warm and moist environment, ideal for their growth.

- In a study, scientists found 1,458 new species of bacteria living just in the bellybutton of human beings. Everyone's belly button ecology is unique, like a fingerprint.

- Some Civil War soldiers had wounds that glowed in the dark because the wounds were infected with bioluminescent bacteria.

- To prove that stomach ulcers were caused by bacteria and not stress, an Australian scientist drank a beaker of the bacterium. He did indeed develop stomach ulcers and won the Nobel Prize in Medicine for his efforts.

- The discoverer of penicillin, Alexander Fleming, warned in the 1920s, soon after penicillin was discovered, about the possibility of antibiotic resistant bacteria due to antibiotics overuse.

- A treatment used for bladder cancer is to inject weakened cow tuberculosis bacteria into the bladder. The immune reaction that this causes destroys the cancer cells.

- Millions of people around the world, especially in East Asia, do not need to use antiperspirants or deodorants as they have a gene that stops them from producing sweat and so they do not attract the bacteria that cause body odour.

- One teaspoon of the bacterium Clostridium botulinum is enough to kill every single person in the USA.

- In 2007, scientists revived an eight-million-year-old bacterium that was extracted from Antarctic ice.

- Antibiotics are often not effective for sore throats and common colds as they are usually caused by viruses rather than bacteria.

WHAT ARE PROBIOTICS?

The reason for talking about bacteria up to this point is that probiotics are usually bacterial. Probiotics are live micro-organisms that, when ingested in adequate amounts, produce a therapeutic or preventive health benefit. The term "probiotics" comes from the Greek words "pro" and "bios" meaning "for" and "life" (as opposed to "antibiotics," which kill bacteria, this term means "against life").

The World Health Organization defines probiotics as *"live micro-organisms, which when administered in adequate amounts confer a health benefit on the host"*. Each of the descriptors in this phrase is important when deciding if a micro-organism, or a product containing them, can accurately be called a probiotic or not.

- **live micro-organisms** - sometimes we administer micro-organisms that are dead, but which can still confer a health benefit. The best examples are bacterial vaccines for diseases such as anthrax, tuberculosis and pneumococcus.
- **administered** - usually means ingested but probiotics have also been administered in other ways, such as through feeding tubes in people who are unable to eat.
- **adequate amounts** - we will talk about how many bacterial cells are needed when taking a product, but the key point here is not so much the number of bacterial cells that are administered, but the number that make it to the intestines and are still alive at that point.
- **confer a health benefit** - this is the hardest part to demonstrate: a genuine probiotic must improve health and the only way to show this is in medical research studies. In terms of the health benefit, this can either be in the form of treating a disease, or preventing a disease. For example, blue cheese contains many species of bacteria, but there is no evidence (at the moment) that these bacteria confer a health benefit.

As well as probiotics, there are prebiotics and synbiotics. These terms can be quite confusing and so these terms, as well as the terms that have been used above to describe micro-organisms and the gastro-intestinal tract, are defined in the following box.

DEFINITIONS

Bacteria - A member of a large group of unicellular micro-organisms that have cell walls but lack organelles and an organized nucleus.

Microbes - Also known as micro-organisms. A microscopic organism, especially a bacterium, virus, or fungus.

Microbiome - The micro-organisms in a particular environment, e.g. the body or a part of the body.

Gut flora - The micro-organisms that are found naturally in the gastro-intestinal tract.

Pathogen - This is anything that can produce disease, but the term usually refers to a micro-organism that causes disease.

Gastro-intestinal (GI) tract - An organ system responsible for consuming and digesting foodstuffs, absorbing nutrients, and expelling waste. The GI tract consists of the stomach and intestines.

Intestine - Also known as the gut or bowel. In human anatomy, the intestine is the segment of the gastro-intestinal tract extending from the pyloric sphincter of the stomach to the anus.

Probiotics - Live micro-organisms, which when administered in adequate amounts confer a health benefit on the host.

Dysbiosis - When the good and bad bacteria in your body get out of balance. Taking probiotics may help correct this.

Prebiotics - A nondigestible food ingredient that promotes the growth of beneficial micro-organisms in the intestines. Common prebiotics are inulin and oligosaccharides.

Synbiotics - Nutritional supplements combining probiotics and prebiotics in a form of synergism, hence synbiotics.

Antibiotics - A medicine (such as penicillin or its derivatives) that inhibits the growth of, or destroys micro-organisms.

FROM ENEMY TO TREATMENT

So how did bacteria come to be seen as being potentially beneficial for health, after previously thought of as being only potentially harmful? Health claims concerning live micro-organisms in food can be seen as far back as a Persian version of the Old Testament (Genesis 18:8), where it states that *"Abraham owed his longevity to the consumption of sour milk."* And over 2,000 years ago, in 76 BC, the Roman historian Plinius recommended the administration of fermented milk products for treating symptoms of gastroenteritis.

Elie Metchnikoff is credited as being one of the first people to put forward the idea that lactic acid bacteria (LAB) had the potential for providing health benefits. He was a Russian biologist and zoologist who was famous for his pioneering research into the immune system and whose work on phagocytes (a type of white blood cell) won him the Nobel Prize in 1908. In 1907 he said that *"... the dependence of the intestinal microbes on the food makes it possible to adopt measures to modify the flora in our bodies and to replace the harmful microbes by useful microbes"*. He said that eating yoghurt containing lactobacilli bacteria results in a reduction of toxin-producing bacteria in the gut.

Another key figure was a French paediatrician called Henry Tissier. He worked at the famous Pasteur Institute and he identified and undertook research on a potentially important probiotic bacteria called Bifidobacterium, which is found in large amounts in the intestinal flora of breast-fed babies. He demonstrated that the bacteria conferred health benefits when used to treat diarrhoea in babies, and suggested that the mechanism by which it worked was by displacing, or taking over from, the harmful bacteria that were causing the illness.

The term "probiotics" was introduced in 1965 by researchers Lilly and Stillwell to describe *"substances secreted by one micro-organisms which stimulates the growth of another"*. In terms of commercial products, Yakult was the first commercially available probiotic drink, introduced in Japan in 1935. It was manufactured by fermenting a mixture of skimmed milk with a special strain of the bacterium Lactobacillus casei and was invented by the Japanese scientist Minoru ShirotaIt. The next major product to be released was Activia, which was first sold in France in 1987. But it is only really in the last decade that probiotic products have become widespread, with most grocery shops in developed countries selling them and millions of people buying them.

CURRENT KNOWLEDGE & MODERN USE OF PROBIOTICS

As we will see in the next chapter, probiotics are hugely popular, and with good reason. There have been dozens of medical research studies completed over the last few decades and the pace of research is, if anything, increasing. If you search for current clinical trials involving probiotics on the website www.clinicaltrials.gov, there are currently around 700 studies at various stages.

One of the reasons for their popularity is the widespread use of antibiotics. This is not a criticism of these medicines - they have saved literally millions of lives since their discovery and will continue to do so in the near future, if not longer. However, as well as killing the harmful bacteria that they are used for, they also wreak havoc with the complicated gut flora, which as we saw previously, is essential to our health. Maybe this will change in the future with the discovery of new and improved antibiotics, but at the moment, they cannot distinguish between good and bad bacteria. There is widespread acknowledgment that antibiotics are prescribed far more often than is necessary. For example, they do not work at all for viral illnesses such as the common cold, but doctors often prescribe them to patients with colds anyway. The average child in the UK has taken ten courses of antibiotics by the age of 16 years.

There is also a potentially more problematic use of antibiotics, and that is their use in animals. More antibiotics are used on animals than on humans. The World Health Organization (WHO) says more than half of the global production of antibiotics is used on farm animals, mostly in farming pigs and chickens. Around 80% of the antibiotics used in the United States are fed to livestock and their diet contains low doses of antibiotics, which are not there to cure a bacterial illness, but to make the animals grow faster and survive cramped living conditions. These antibiotics may pass through the food chain to humans and affect our gut flora.

As well as antibiotics, other aspects of modern living may be contributing to a reduction in the proportion of "good" bacteria, which should be around 10-15% of the bacteria in the gut in adults. A poor diet, such as one that contains too much fatty, low fibre, preservative-laden food, environmental factors such as pollution and even stress have all been linked to a reduction in beneficial gut bacteria.

The remainder of this book summarises our current knowledge of probiotics, describes the medical research evidence for various medical conditions for which they are commonly used, addresses issues of safety and in the next chapter, gives an overview of the myriad of different products that are available.

Chapter 2

PRODUCTS

Probiotic products contain billions of bacteria, but it can also seem that there are millions of products to choose from. There are different formulations (such as yoghurts, capsules and drinks), different bacteria in the products, different amounts of the bacteria in the products and also sometimes different additional components in the products (such as enteric coating or prebiotics). This chapter looks at all these different options, so that if and when you choose a take a probiotic product you will know exactly what to look for when making your choice.

BILLIONS OF BUGS, BILLIONS OF DOLLARS

With the recent huge increase in the potential health benefits of probiotics, they have moved from a niche complementary medicine to being an enormous industry in their own right. Annual global sales of probiotics are predicted to rise to US$42 billion by 2016. The market is predicted to grow by an estimated US$120 million......every month! In the UK alone, 3.5 million people take probiotic supplements in some form daily. Some regions have increased their use by even more than the average, particularly Eastern Europe, Asia Pacific and Latin America - nearly half of all probiotics sold globally in 2014 were in these regions. Overall, the largest consumers of probiotics in 2014 were Western Europe followed by Asia Pacific, Japan, Latin America, North America and then Eastern Europe.

Reasons for this rapid growth include:

- The publication of hundreds of medical research papers every year, many showing positive health benefits.
- A surge in stories about probiotics in newspapers, magazines and on TV, meaning that people are much more aware of the potential benefits.

- Readily accessible information being available on the internet. Health topics are the second most commonly searched for items on search engines.
- An increasing acknowledgement of the potential benefits of probiotics by doctors and other health professionals, many of whom now recommend them for certain conditions.

Also, in general, over the last few decades we have seen a rapid increase in interest in natural, complementary and alternative medicines and therapies. Many reasons have been put forward for this including a general distrust of government health systems, the exponentially rising cost of modern healthcare, difficulty accessing healthcare and disillusionment with some or many aspects of modern medicine, such as a perceived focus on prescribing medicines (often with side effects) to treat symptoms, rather than focusing on preventing diseases occurring in the first place. Overall, we have seen moves away from being told what to do by health professionals, towards taking more responsibility for our own health and treatments and also away from treating illnesses after they occur to preventing them in the first place. The increasing use of probiotics to prevent ill health fits perfectly into this paradigm shift.

AND HUNDREDS OF PRODUCTS

When it comes to choosing a probiotic product we are spoiled for choice. A number of formats are available and this choice is useful, as some people may prefer a food or drink, others may prefer to swallow a pill or capsule. There are no main advantages or disadvantages of one format over another, it is simply a case of consumer preference. Overall, many people are not very good at taking medicines or health supplements on a regular basis long-term, as would be required if taking probiotics daily as a health supplement to prevent or treat illnesses. An important element in achieving a high level of adherence (i.e. missing very few doses of a product) is having a format that you are happy with, so the variety of formats that probiotics are available in is very useful.

Foods - Many foods contain live bacteria and other micro-organisms, particularly fermented foods. Fermentation is the process in which a substance, usually a sugar or starch, breaks down into a simpler substance. Micro-organisms like yeast and bacteria usually play a role in the fermentation process, creating beer, wine, bread and yoghurt to name just a few. However, as we discussed previously when we defined what a probiotic is, we saw that being a live micro-organisms is not enough, it also needs to both survive the journey down the gastro-intestinal tract to the intestines and confer a health benefit.

It is often assumed that eating yoghurt will give a person all the probiotics they need, but care needs to be taken when choosing a product. Some yoghurts are pasteurized, which kills the bacteria; however all may not be lost as some of these yoghurts have live cultures added back in after the pasteurization process. The yoghurt needs to say "live" or "active cultures" on the label to potentially be a probiotic. Ideally it would say "probiotic" and contain them in sufficient quantities, but unfortunately many types of yoghurt are mislabelled as containing probiotics when they do not.

In the USA, the National Yoghurt Association has introduced a "Live Active Culture Seal" to identify refrigerated or frozen yoghurt products that contain at least a minimum number of viable lactic acid bacteria per gram at the time of manufacture. The milk used to make yoghurt can come from any animal such as a goat, sheep or cow.

There is no reason why probiotics cannot be added to many foods, and a number of such probiotic-fortified foods are available. Examples include a cornflake cereal which also contains coin drops of yoghurt that deliver Lactobacillus acidophilus, and a company called Attune sells granola and chocolate bars which contain a blend of three probiotics. In 2006, a New Orleans entrepreneur started a company called Naked Pizza which sold pies made with probiotic-enriched crust!

Another food product that is gaining in popularity is kefir. This is similar to yoghurt but is 99% lactose free, making it a good option for those who are lactose intolerant. It has around three times the amount of probiotics that are typically found in yoghurt.

Finally with respect to foods, there are two traditional foods that contain live bacteria which are claimed to confer health benefits. One of these is *miso* which is a traditional Japanese food and medicine made from fermented rye, beans, rice or barley. The other common one is *sauerkraut*, most commonly associated with Germany, which is made from fermented cabbage (and sometimes other vegetables).

Drinks - Many people around the world start their day with a probiotic drink. Popular brands include Align, Biobalance, Bio-Kult and Probio 7. The most famous are probably Yakult, made by the Japanese company of the same name, and Actimel, made by French company Danone. They are usually dairy-based beverages with a consistency similar to milk, some manufacturers describe their probiotic drinks as drinkable yoghurts.

Capsules/Tablets - finally, probiotics are also available as capsules or tablets to be swallowed whole, or it is possible to buy the probiotic powder that they contain, which can be added to water or a smoothie, or sprinkled on any cold food.

WHICH BUG?

As discussed above, not all bacteria are probiotics: they have to both be able to colonize the gut, and attach to its lining, after having survived the journey through the strongly acidic stomach AND confer a proven health benefit. Although there are thousands of bacteria and millions of other micro-organisms, because of these requirements, there are not many probiotics. With more research it is almost certain that many more probiotic micro-organisms will be discovered, probably a number every year, but at the moment we only know of several dozen and most of these are strains from what is known as the Lactic acid family of bacteria.

Before we go any further it is necessary to understand the way in which bacteria are named, and an analogy that is commonly used is useful here. We all know that Germany makes cars, Volkswagen is a manufacturer of some cars in Germany, one of the cars they make is the VW Golf, and that there are a number of different models of the VW Golf with different specifications, such as the VW Golf 1.4D. Applying a similar breakdown to a common probiotic: the bacterial family of these probiotic bacteria is the lactic acid bacteria, the genus is Lactobacillus, the species is Lactobacillus acidophilus and the strain is Lactobacillus acidophilus LC1. And so the strain of a bacteria is the equivalent of the make and model of a car. The key point to be aware of is that when we discuss the effectiveness of probiotics for certain conditions, based on the medical research, the research only applies to the exact strain that was tested. In our analogy, this means that the results of testing a car only apply to that particular make and model. If a VW Golf 1.4D is tested and it travels 100km/litre of fuel, or has a top speed of 140km/hour, you cannot say that a VW Beetle 2015 will have the same fuel efficiency or top speed. It might do, but you would have to test this exact make and model before making any claims.

NAMING CARS AND BACTERIA		
German car	Bacterial family	Lactic acid bacteria
Volkswagen	Bacterial genus	Lactobacillus
VW Golf	Bacterial species	Lactobacillus acidophilus
VW Golf 1.4D	Bacterial strain	Lactobacillus acidophilus LC1

A table of the main probiotic micro-organisms is provided below, and in chapters four and five we will discuss the actual and potential medical benefits of different probiotics. However, one aspect to be aware of at this stage is that many of the currently known probiotics and much of the completed and ongoing medical research into probiotics, are from the Lactic acid bacteria family. Further, many of the currently known probiotics are strains of two particular genus of Lactic acid bacteria: Lactobacillus and Bifidobacterium. Just one of the probiotics is not a bacteria: Saccharomyces cerevisiae is a yeast.

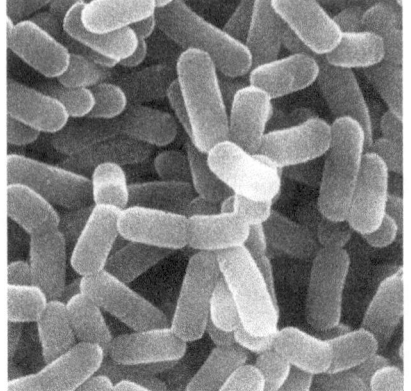
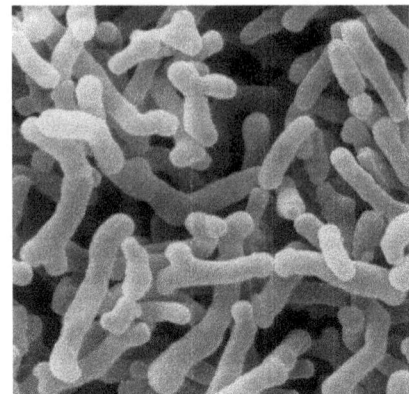

Lactobacillus casei *Bifidobacterium bacteria*

As you can see in the picture, Lactobacillus are rod-shaped bacteria. They convert lactose and other sugars to lactic acid and play a beneficial role in the body on the whole, the exception being in the mouth where they are associated with cavities and tooth decay. Part of the mechanism by which they act as probiotics is that the production of lactic acid makes their immediate environment acidic and this can help to inhibit the growth of some harmful bacteria. The popular Yakult drink contains a strain of the probiotic bacterium Lactobacillus casei Shirota.

The other major probiotic genus are the Bifidobacterium bacteria, and as you can see from the picture, they often have a distinctive branched shape. Activia, a brand of yoghurt owned and marketed by global giant Danone, contains the probiotic Bifidobacterium animalis DN 173,010.

GENUS	PROBIOTIC SPECIES
Lactobacillus (Commonly abbreviated to L.)	L. acidophilus, L. casei, L. bulgaricus, L. fermentum, L. thermophilus, L. rhamnosus, L. casei, L. caucasicus, L. helveticus, L. lactis, L. reuteri, L. plantarum, L. brevis, L. johnsonii
Bifidobacterium (Commonly abbreviated to B.)	B. longum, B. bifidum, B. infantis, B. animalis, B. lactis
Escherichia	Escherichia coli
Bacillus	Bacillus cereus, Bacillus clausii, Bacillus pumilus
Propionibacterium	Propionibacterium freudenreichii
Enterococcus	Enterococcus faecium
Streptococcus	Streptococcus thermophilus, Streptococcus cremoris, Streptococcus faecium, Streptococcus infantis
Saccharomyces (yeast)	Saccharomyces cerevisiae, Saccharomyces boulardii

Probiotic products contain either a single probiotic strain, or a blend of several different strains. Studies have not proven if a blend of different strains is better than a single one, but it is certainly feasible that this may be the case, particularly if probiotics are being taken as a general health supplement rather than to treat or prevent a specific disease.

HOW MANY?

In order to work, probiotic microbes need to survive the journey down the gastro-intestinal tract all the way from the mouth to the intestines, without dying along the way. In fact they have to survive a lot more than that before they even get to your mouth; they have to survive the manufacturing processes and also the time that they spend sitting on a shelf in a shop waiting for you to buy them and then in your medicine cabinet.

DEFINITION OF CFU

CFUs stands for "colony-forming units" and is the way in which the number of probiotic microbes is measured and described. It is an estimate of the number of "viable" bacteria or fungal cells in a sample. Viable is defined as the ability to multiply. There are both manual and automated systems for determining the number of CFUs in a sample. The number of microbes could also be estimated by simply looking at a sample down a microscope, but this would result in a count that included both living and the dead microbes.

Therefore, the dose of a probiotic, instead of a number of milligrams or grams as we would use for a medicine in a tablet, is the number of cells or CFUs. We will discuss specific doses that have been tested in studies in Chapters four and five, but in general, doses of probiotics are in the range of one to 10 billion cells / day. Lower doses are likely to be ineffective, and higher doses are safe, but probably not necessary and therefore expensive as consumers would be paying for extra probiotics that they do not need. Unfortunately, as we will see in the next section, the number of cells in a dose of a product may not be accurate.

QUALITY OF PROBIOTIC PRODUCTS

Quality control problems are unfortunately common with many natural products and probiotics are no exception. There is the issue of contamination, when products contain components that are not listed on the label and may even be harmful, an example being mercury and other heavy metal contamination of omega-3 fish oil products. A bigger issue though is that some natural product supplements do not contain or deliver the full dose that it is stated in the label and this is a particular problem for probiotics. Even if the manufacturer attempts to have the correct number of cells in the product, and the product has the correct number of live cells when it leaves the factory, what matters to the consumer is whether the product contains the correct number of live cells when they actually consume the product. Manufacturers should factor in that a lot of cells will die over time and so they need to make sure that at the end of the shelf-life of the product, it delivers at least the number of live cells as is stated on the label. Companies may therefore produce probiotic products with around double the number of labelled live cells, having determined that around half will die before the expiry date. (Do not worry about these dead cells, they are not harmful, it's just that they will not be helpful).

Testing undertaken by ConsumerLab.com in 2012 of probiotic products found that some products had far lower amounts of live cells than was claimed on the label. However, all of the products tested provided at least one billion organisms per day.

Manufacturers sometimes modify the products in order to make sure that the cells stay alive during storage and during the passage down the gastro-intestinal tract. For example, some probiotic tablet and capsule products have an enteric-coating — this a polymer barrier that is added to the tablet or capsule, and protects it from the strong acidity of the stomach. Another modification is the addition of prebiotics to the product. Prebiotics are usually types of sugar and you can think of them as food for the probiotics microbes, to keep them healthy and alive until they reach your intestines. This combination of prebiotic and probiotic is referred to as a *symbiotic* product. A novel and effective way to deliver symbiotic products is a "capsule in a capsule", whereby the probiotic bacteria are enclosed in a small inner capsule, which is then placed inside another capsule which is filled with the prebiotic.

What can you do to make sure that you are getting a sufficient number of cells, other than setting up your own laboratory to test products yourself? The main things you can do are; buy from a reputable manufacturer that you have heard of; consider a product with an enteric-coat or with added prebiotics; store the products as instructed on the label (for example, many but not all probiotic products require refrigeration); and use the products before they expire (literally!).

Chapter 3
HOW THEY WORK

We have discussed what probiotics are (and what they are not), and also what types of products are available. In the next two chapters we will cover which medical conditions people take them for and look at the research evidence for their effectiveness. Without giving too much away, probiotics tend to be taken for a wide range of health issues, but these can be neatly divided into health problems and diseases of the gastro-intestinal tract (covered in chapter four) and health problems and diseases *outside of* the gastro-intestinal tract (covered in chapter five).

We saw earlier that probiotics are taken into the body via the mouth (or rarely a nasal feeding tube) and pass through the gastro-intestinal tract into the intestines. They do not get absorbed into the bloodstream and travel around the body to other organs - they pass out of the body in the same way that anything else you eat and do not absorb passes out - in the faeces. To satisfy the definition of a probiotic they have to be alive in the intestines in sufficient numbers to confer a health benefit, and this is where they live, until, like any organism, they die and leave the body. As they live in the intestines, it is easy to see how they may help with health problems and diseases of the gastro-intestinal tract, such as diarrhoea and irritable bowel syndrome. Many people only take them for bowel-related problems and may not be aware that there are other very different potential uses. It is harder to see how they can be useful for diseases that do not involve the intestines, such as boosting the immune system, alleviating allergic conditions such as eczema or even preventing cancer, but many people take them for these and other reasons and the evidence is discussed in Chapter five. The remainder of this chapter discusses how probiotics are thought to work and confer health benefits and like all subjects of medical research, our knowledge is growing rapidly, with important new information being published in medical journals and at scientific conferences, even while this book was being written!

There are three main mechanisms by which probiotics act in the body that can lead to effects on health:

1. COMPETITIVE EXCLUSION OF OTHER BACTERIA

We will start with the easiest to understand of the three main mechanisms. You go to the shopping mall late on Christmas Eve and there is nowhere for you to park your car because all the spaces have been taken by other frantic shoppers. It's the same for the linings of the intestines - once bacteria have attached themselves to the wall of the intestines, it is very hard for other bacteria to displace them. You will recall how, earlier we said that a good dose of probiotics was one to 10 billion cells per day and this is the reason why....the idea is that there are many more of the good bacteria (the probiotic bacteria) than the bad ones that either do not improve health or worse, actually harm health, in the intestines. Then, when parking spots on the intestine walls become available, the odds are that the good ones will lodge there. This process of attaching and then hopefully living and multiplying in an area is called "colonisation". It's a tough life for the bacteria - they compete for spaces on the intestine walls and those that colonise will thrive and exclude others, hence the term "competitive colonisation". One of the key characteristics of probiotics as opposed to other bacteria, is that they by definition must have an excellent ability to adhere and bind to the intestine wall.

It is not just space that the probiotics fight for, they also fight for nutrients. Probiotics and other bacteria compete for essential nutrients, and the losers in this race will die. Using our shopping mall analogy, as well as fighting for parking spaces, they also fight for items in the shops as well.

These concepts of competition and exclusion are what most people think of when they think of how probiotics work. In simple terms, which are also accurate, the aim in taking probiotics is to replace bad bacteria with good ones.

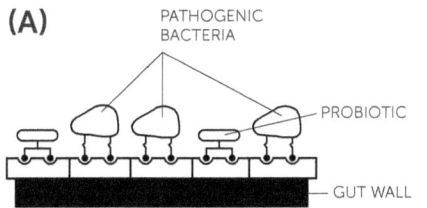 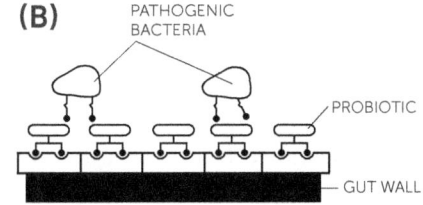

2. ANTIBACTERIAL ACTIONS

The second main mechanism by which probiotic bacteria act is to actually attack and kill other bacteria; again, either those bacteria which do not improve health or those which actually harm health. There are at least three main ways in which this can occur:

i) Production of antibacterial substances.

We are all familiar with antibiotic medications, medicines that we take when we have bacterial infections such as a chest infection. One of the most famous is of course penicillin, which was discovered by accident in 1928 by Alexander Fleming. Legend has it that he noticed a Petri dish containing Staphylococcus bacteria, that had mistakenly been left open, was contaminated by blue-green mould which had entered the laboratory from an open window. Fleming observed that there was an area with none of the Staphylococcus bacteria in a ring around this mould, and rightly concluded that the mould had produced and released a substance that had either killed or at least stopped the growth of the bacteria.

What you may not realize though is that many antibiotics which kill bacteria, such as penicillin, are actually made by other bacteria! We have already discussed above how bacteria compete against each other and one of the ways is by direct chemical warfare; they produce a range of chemicals that can kill their bacterial cousins. The chemicals they can produce include hydrogen peroxide, a naturally-occurring form of bleach, organic acids, and other chemicals that can kill bacteria (collectively known as bacteriocins). Disease-causing (i.e. pathogenic) bacteria that probiotic bacteria can attack with chemicals include

Escherichia coli, Clostridium difficile and Salmonella species. The diseases that these bacteria can cause are discussed in more detail in the next chapter. The shopping mall car park analogy is again useful to illustrate this concept of antibacterial actions...this time, the people are getting out of their cars and attacking each other!

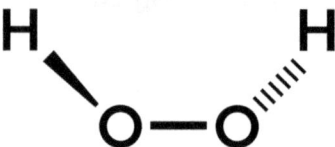

Hydrogen Peroxide

ii) Lowering luminal pH

A slightly more subtle way by which probiotics can fight off other bacteria is by actively changing the environment of the intestines so that it favours their survival and harms the chances of survival for their enemies. As discussed, they can produce chemicals including hydrogen peroxide and organic acids. These lower the pH of the space within the intestines (the lumen) i.e. make it more acidic. One of the key acids that is released is lactic acid, produced as you would guess by the Lactobacillus family of bacteria. These include the many Lactobacillus and Bifidobacterium species that are used as probiotics and some of the key (but not essential) characteristics of a bacteria that make it a potential probiotic is the ability to produce acids and to thrive in an acidic environment.

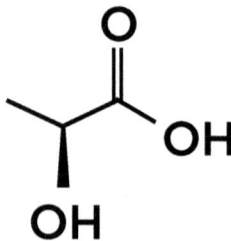

Lactic Acid

iii) Degradation of toxin receptor

Finally with respect to mechanisms by which probiotics adversely affect competing bacteria, is a slightly different method that is used in some situations and can be very effective. Rather than fighting the bad bacteria directly, with acids and other chemicals, some probiotics can stop the bad bacteria from causing their harmful effects without directly affecting the bad bacteria themselves. The best example is Clostridium difficile infection. We will discuss this in more detail in the next chapter, but it is a bacteria which causes a particularly nasty and dangerous type of diarrhoea. It does this by releasing a toxin, the toxin binds to receptors on the gastro-intestinal wall cells and this causes inflammation and diarrhoea. The probiotic bacteria Streptococcus boulardii is thought to prevent this particular infection by degrading (destroying) these receptors and therefore prevents the infection without directly harming the C. difficile bacteria.

3. MODIFYING THE IMMUNE SYSTEM

The role of the immune system is to defend us against disease-causing micro-organisms, so when it is working well we have better health by having fewer infections. However, it can also cause some illnesses if it is not working properly, particularly by being too active and fighting things in our environment that are not dangerous (e.g. fighting pollen and causing hay-fever, or fighting the body's own structures in rheumatoid arthritis). It is formally defined as *"...a system of biological structures and processes within an organism that protects against disease."* In simple terms, it consists of barriers and cells/chemicals. The **barriers** include:

- physical barriers - such as the skin or gastro-intestinal tract,
- chemical barriers - such as stomach acid,
- microbial barriers - friendly bacteria that live in the body as discussed above, or are taken into the body when we have probiotics.

There are hundreds if not thousands of cells and chemicals involved in the immune system, with millions of interactions

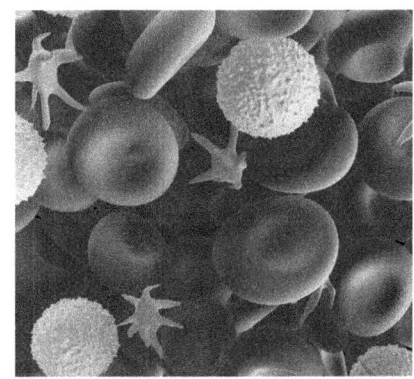

Blood cells

occurring. We will not go into this in any more detail, except to say that most of this activity is mediated by different types of white blood cells such as neutrophils, monocytes, eosinophils and basophils.

The important message here is that around 70% of the body's immune cells live in the gastro-intestinal tract. Probiotics have been shown to influence the immune system in the gastro-intestinal tract in a number of ways and thereby make it more effective, i.e. they can give a boost to your immune system. These influences include:

- Increasing the number of gastro-intestinal cells that produce and release immunoglobulins (antibodies).
- Helping to speed up the immune reaction to disease-causing bacteria.
- Producing chemicals that strengthen the gastro-intestinal cells' barriers against pathogen invasion.

The immune system is hugely important to our health, and we can see this in the devastating consequences that are seen when it is not working well, e.g. in people with HIV infection or leukemia. It has only recently become understood that micro-organisms in the body play such an important role in the immune system. This is one of the main reasons why people take probiotics and researchers are looking for and finding real health benefits from taking them.

Chapter 4

GASTRO-INTESTINAL DISEASES

After learning what probiotics are, what to look for when buying products and how they work, it's now time to see which conditions they work for. There are a few important points to bear in mind when we look at the various conditions and the supporting evidence below. Even though I'll be giving a rating for the effectiveness of probiotics for each condition, this is not my opinion I am giving you! Instead, it is an assessment of what the research that has been done says. Also, as much as possible, I'll be looking at all the relevant research studies that have been done. I've lost count of the times that people have sent me a copy of a positive research study and claimed that it is proof that a product works for a certain condition, but they did not know about (or tell me about) the 20 studies that found just the opposite and showed that the product was not effective. In research, we acknowledge that sometimes even well-conducted studies may not give the real answer, and up to 5% of the time a positive study may have given the wrong result due to chance. This is why an initial positive trial should always be repeated. When a person selectively quotes a single positive study and ignores the many negative ones, this is called "cherry-picking".

Also at this stage it would be useful to define how the word "significant" is used in terms of medical research findings, as it is often misunderstood or used incorrectly. The reason for the confusion is that there are two common ways that the word is used, which have very different meanings. "*Clinical significance*" means that the size of the effect of a treatment is of such a magnitude that it is important and will affect health. For example, a decrease in systolic blood pressure from 150 to 100 mm Hg is highly likely to have health benefits and so this reduction can accurately be said to be clinically significant. "*Statistical significance*" however means that the result of a clinical trial is unlikely to have occurred by chance and, without delving too deeply into the complex world of statistics, this usually means that there is a 95% likelihood that the result of the trial is actually the true result, i.e. there is only a 5% chance that the result of the trial may be incorrect. Statistical significance is closely related to the number of subjects in the research study, as the larger the study, the more likely its results will be the true result.

Another important point to remember is that the information in this book is correct at the time of writing, in 2015. New research on probiotics is being reported every week and it is certainly possible that in the future some may be shown not to be effective for some conditions that we currently think they work for. It is also very likely that new research findings will show probiotics to be effective for conditions that we do not think they are effective for at the moment.

With these points in mind, each condition that we will be looking at will have a rating, as follows:

RATING SYSTEM

* very little or no good evidence of effectiveness

** small amount of evidence of effectiveness

*** moderate amount of evidence of effectiveness

**** very good evidence of effectiveness

Diarrhoea

**** very good evidence of effectiveness

Diarrhoea occurs when a person has bowel movements (stools) that are described as loose and watery. It is very common, with the average person experiencing symptoms once or twice a year and is very rarely serious. It usually lasts for two to three days unless it is associated with an underlying medical condition such as irritable bowel syndrome. The most common cause is a virus that infects the GI tract, and for this reason it is sometimes (incorrectly) called "intestinal flu" or "stomach flu." Other causes include infection by bacteria (i.e. food poisoning), eating certain foods, allergies to certain foods, a side effect of some medications, medical treatments such as radiation therapy and other diseases of the GI tract. In this section, we will be discussing acute diarrhoea (i.e. quite sudden onset and a short duration) usually due to a virus, bacteria or food poisoning and some specific forms of diarrhoea are discussed later in the chapter. This form of diarrhoea is defined by the World Health Organization (WHO) as three or more loose or watery stools in a 24-hour period, with the symptoms starting less than 14 days previously.

As well as loose and watery stools, other symptoms can include abdominal bloating or cramps, nausea or vomiting. Rare but serious symptoms are blood or mucus in the stools, weight loss or fever. The vast majority of cases are mild, self-limiting and the only thing a person needs to do is be meticulous in washing their hands, so that it is not transmitted to others, and drink plenty of fluids.

While in Western countries the illness is more of a nuisance than a danger, the same cannot be said for developing countries. In these areas children usually have six to 12 episodes per year, compared with around two per year in developed countries. It causes around two million deaths per year in low- and middle-income countries, mostly in children under five years of age.

More than 20 micro-organisms (viruses, bacteria and parasites) are known to frequently cause acute diarrhoea. The most prevalent is rotavirus, the bacteria that can be responsible include Escherichia coli, Salmonella, Shigella, Yersinia, Campylobacter and Vibrio cholerae.

The main parasitic causes of diarrhoea are Cryptosporidium and Giardia. However, in most cases we do not know and never find out the actual micro-organism that is responsible for a particular episode.

This topic has been covered in a Cochrane Review. These reviews, as defined by the Cochrane Collaboration website (http://community.cochrane.org/) are defined as *"... systematic reviews of primary research in human health care and health policy, and are internationally recognised as the highest standard in evidence-based health care."*

These review are conducted by experts in analysing scientific research, and as they look at all the research around a medical issue independently, many people (including myself) consider these reviews to be the highest form of medical research evidence. Therefore Cochrane Reviews will be discussed in this book if they have looked at the topic, if they have not, then a similar review will be looked at. If this is not available, then individual studies on the topic will be discussed and assessed.

The review included all relevant studies which compared a specified probiotic with a placebo, or no probiotic, in people with acute diarrhoea which was proven to be, or at least presumed to be, caused by an infectious agent. A placebo resembles a pill or another form of medicine but does not actually contain any real medicine. The reason they are used in trials is because of the placebo effect - a medical condition can improve if someone believes that they are taking an effective treatment. This is a poorly understood but definitely real phenomenon and by having a group of people taking placebo in a clinical trial, we can show, hopefully, that the treatment that we are testing actually works and it is not just the placebo effect.

63 studies were included in the analysis that was undertaken as part of this review, the total number of people involved was over 8,000. Interestingly and appropriately, 56 of the 63 trials enrolled infants and young children, only seven involved adults.

The results of the review were overwhelmingly positive. For the main outcomes that were assessed, probiotics:

- reduced the mean duration of diarrhoea by an average of around 25 hours.
- reduced the number of times diarrhoea lasted for four or more days.
- reduced stool frequency.

The authors of the review described the results as "striking", in that almost all of the studies were positive.

As the studies used many different types and amounts of probiotics, the review tried to look at which strain/amount was the best. No firm conclusions could be drawn, with a number of probiotics being shown to be effective, including: Lactobacillus casei strain GG, L. delbrueckii, L. acidophilus, Streptococcus thermophilus, Bacillus bifidum, Streptococcus boulardii, L. rhamnosus, Bifidobacterium lactis B12, L. reuteri. The probiotic strains that were used in more studies than others and therefore have the best evidence to support their use, were Lactobacillus rhamnosus casei GG (LGG) and Bifidobacterium lactis BB-12. As few studies involved adults, it was not possible to see if there was a difference in effectiveness between adults and children. Neither did the studies help to determine the number of organisms needed to be effective – as a wide range of doses were used and most of the studies were positive regardless of dose. An analysis comparing studies with a dose of less than 10 billion, to studies using a dose of more than 10 billion found little difference. There was almost no difference in effectiveness when the researchers compared probiotic products containing a single bacteria product compared to those containing two or more bacteria.

Prevention of diarrhoea / Traveller's diarrhoea

**** very good evidence of effectiveness

So we have seen that probiotics are very effective at treating infectious diarrhoea, but can they stop it occurring in the first place? There is one situation where most people half-expect to get diarrhoea, and that is when they are traveling overseas. Traveller's diarrhoea (TD) is the name of this condition and its incidence (i.e. a measure of the probability of a disease occurring) varies depending on where you are travelling to. In parts of northern Africa, Latin America, the Middle East and Southeast Asia there is a very high incidence, and you would have over 50% of people suffering from TD on your trip. At the lower end of the range, the incidence can be as low as 5–10% of people traveling to countries such as North America, Northern Europe, Australia, New Zealand and the United Kingdom.

Why do we tend to get diarrhoea when we travel overseas? Many aspects of travel such as stress, jet lag, unfamiliar foods and water and disrupted body rhythms can all disturb the normally protective bacteria in our intestines, making us more susceptible to infections. Then on top of this, TD occurs when we eat or drink faecally contaminated food, water or other liquids. Items that we consume that are potentially higher-risk include: raw or undercooked meats and seafood, unpeeled raw fruits and vegetables, tap water, ice, unpasteurized milk and other dairy products. Food and drink from street vendors, farmers' markets and small restaurants are particularly high-risk potential sources of TD. As well as individual travellers, outbreaks of TD can occur in large groups of travellers, one of the best examples being passengers on cruise ships, who can be struck down by the infamous norovirus.

The time from exposure to the contaminated food or liquid to the beginning of symptoms (i.e. the incubation period) is usually two to three days. Diarrhoea is of course the main symptom, typically lasting for two to six days, and can even contain blood in severe cases. Other common symptoms are abdominal cramps, nausea and vomiting, fever and rarely, prolonged diarrhoea for up to one year. The cause in most cases, is a toxic product made by a bacteria (i.e. a pathogen). The most common bacteria that can produce these pathogens are types of Escherichia coli, Bacillus cereus, Clostridium botulinum and Staphylococcus aureus.

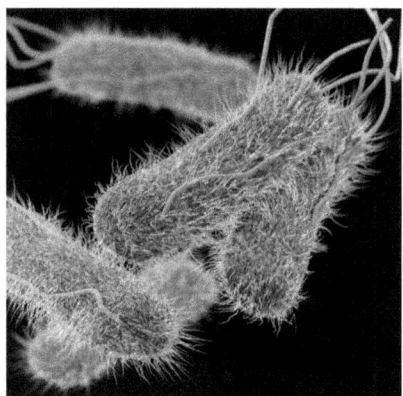
Salmonella

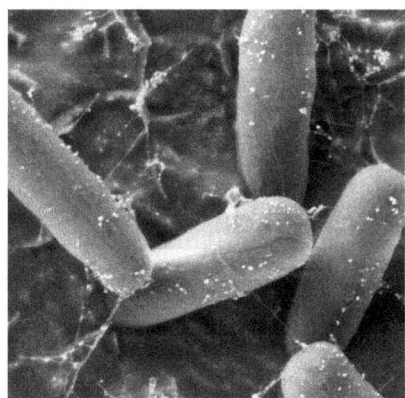
Escherichia coli

The best thing a traveller can do to avoid getting TD is to avoid contaminated foods and liquids, although this can be very hard, if not impossible. In terms of standard medical treatments, the best advice is to simply stay hydrated by drinking lots of non-contaminated water e.g. bottled water. Some people take prophylactic (a medicine or course of action used to prevent disease) antibiotics but this is not generally recommended for several reasons:

- Studies show that they are not very effective, as antibiotics tend to work against specific bacteria. TD can be caused by a wide range of bacteria and also by many viruses and parasites that are not bacteria and therefore would not be killed by antibiotics anyway.
- It contributes to the global health threat of antibiotic resistance.
- Antibiotics, as we will see in a section below, often cause diarrhoea themselves anyway!

There is something that you can do though and not surprisingly, probiotics could be the answer since, as have we have discussed above, amongst other actions they can inhibit pathogen attachment, enhancing the immune response and assist in re-establishing normal microflora.

A review paper has looked at all the good studies on the use of probiotics for the prevention of traveller's diarrhoea. The study authors found 12 studies that they could include in the review, and these studies enrolled between them a total of 4,709 people. When the results of these 12 trials were added together, they showed that probiotics are very effective and the researchers estimated that 85% of TD cases were prevented by probiotics. Several different probiotics were used in the studies and the products that showed the most effectiveness were Saccharomyces boulardii and a mixture of Lactobacillus acidophilus and Bifidobacterium bifidum. In the trials, participants were told to take the probiotics during the whole trip and the trips ranged from eight days to three weeks.

Therefore, as you can have over a 50% chance of getting TD, which could at the least inconvenience you and at worse, ruin the whole trip, and as probiotics reduce the chance of this by 85%, they are strongly recommended and should be the second thing you pack...after your passport!

Antibiotic-Associated Diarrhoea (AAD)

**** very good evidence of effectiveness

The World Health Organisation defines antibiotic-associated diarrhoea (AAD) as three or more abnormally loose bowel movements per 24 hours while on antibiotics. As we have seen, there are over 500 different species of micro-organisms residing in the GI tract and when antibiotics are taken, a large proportion of the beneficial micro-organisms resident in the gut become disrupted. This leads to an increased vulnerability to colonisation of the gut by pathogenic bacteria, and an increased risk of developing an intestinal infection, with the main symptom being diarrhoea. In other words, the antibiotic can kill off our normal "good" bacteria and "bad" bacteria can thrive as a result. As well as the obvious unpleasantness of a bout of diarrhoea, the person who was prescribed the course of antibiotics, for obvious reasons, may decide not to complete the course of antibiotics if they attribute GI side effects to the drug. There are two major downsides to this scenario: the bacterial infection that the person had that was being treated with antibiotics may not be fully treated if the course of antibiotics is shortened; also, not completing the course of antibiotics can leave some of those disease-causing bacteria alive and strengthened, as exposure to antibiotics without being killed can help a bacteria develop resistance to the antibiotic.

Up to 40% of adults who take a course of antibiotics suffer from acute diarrhoea, which can in some cases, lead to chronic or persistent diarrhoea. It is estimated that 25% of cases of AAD are caused by Clostridium difficile which can lead to a particularly nasty and dangerous form of bowel inflammation called colitis, particularly in elderly hospital inpatients. The incidence of diarrhoea in children receiving broad spectrum antibiotics has been reported to be in the range of 11-40%.

There have been a large number of excellent studies that have looked at the use of probiotics to prevent AAD in adults, children and also specifically if they can prevent the dangerous Clostridium difficile diarrhoea.

For adults, a systematic review and meta-analysis of the use of probiotics for the prevention and treatment AAD was published in *JAMA, the Journal of the American Medical Association,* in 2012. 63 studies with 11,811 participants were included in the analysis and the main finding was that probiotic use was associated with a much lower risk of developing diarrhoea, compared with people in the studies who were not using probiotics. Overall, the chances of getting ADD are reduced by 42%. The usual probiotics, often Lactobacillus-based were tested in the various studies, and the researchers determined that none of the species or combinations showed substantial superiority over the others.

As for children, a Cochrane Review of probiotics for the prevention of paediatric AAD was published in 2007. There were fewer studies in children, ten clinical trials were identified, involving a total of just under 2,000 children. Six of the ten trials used lactic acid bacteria probiotics and the results were actually better than in adults, with an average reduction in the chance of getting AAD of 51%.

Finally, a Cochrane Review of probiotics for the prevention of Clostridium difficile-associated diarrhoea (CDAD) in adults and children was published in 2013. In this review, 31 trials which enrolled 4,492 participants were included in this analysis. The results were even better again, with the main finding being that when probiotics are given with antibiotics, they reduce the risk of developing CDAD by 64%.

These results are quite remarkable and worth repeating. Up to 40% of people get diarrhoea with antibiotics, and around a quarter of the time it is the nasty Clostridium difficile variety. Taking a couple of weeks of inexpensive and safe probiotics reduces the chances of this by nearly a half in adults, a half in children and for the Clostridium difficile variety by around two thirds!

There is a practical point to be aware of when taking probiotics with antibiotics to treat or prevent AAD. Firstly, it is advisable to stagger the administration of the antibiotic and probiotic so that the probiotic is administered at least two hours after the antibiotic dose, where possible, otherwise the antibiotic may reduce the efficacy of the probiotic micro-organisms by killing them. Fortunately, and importantly, the reverse is not

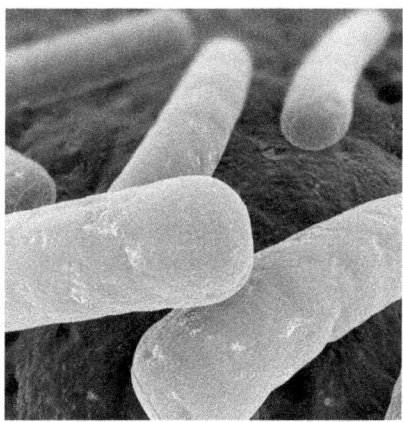

Clostridium difficile

true: probiotics will not cause a reduction in the effectiveness of the antibiotic. As to how long the course of probiotics should be, there is less certainty on this from the medical literature, with one-three weeks being standard in the trials, overall it appears that a two-week course is sufficient. As most courses of antibiotics are for five to ten days, this means continuing for a few days after the antibiotics have finished, and hence repopulating the GI tract with the healthy bacteria.

A few years ago this author was one of the first researchers to advocate the use of probiotics with antibiotics and predicted that soon almost all doctors would recommend a course of probiotics when they reach for their prescription pad and write down instructions for a course of antibiotics. This is proving to be correct; more and more doctors are doing this, and soon it is likely to be the norm, with probiotics moving from a fringe concept, only popular amongst people with a big interest in natural health and complementary therapies, to a routine part of mainstream medicine.

Radiation-induced diarrhoea

*** moderate amount of evidence of effectiveness

To conclude our look at different types of diarrhoea, people who have had cancer and as part of their treatment have had radiation therapy are often affected by troublesome diarrhoea. Radiotherapy is the use of high-energy rays, which are usually x-rays, to treat diseases, particularly cancers that are in the abdomen or pelvis areas. It works by destroying cancer cells in the area that is treated and although normal non-cancerous cells can also be damaged by the radiotherapy, these cells can usually repair themselves, but the cancer cells cannot. According to the NHS in the UK, almost half of all people with cancer have radiotherapy as part of their treatment plan. Radiotherapy can be given in two different ways – from outside the body (external radiotherapy, whereby a machine focuses high-energy radiation beams onto the area requiring treatment) or inside the body (internal radiotherapy, whereby a small piece of radioactive material is placed temporarily inside the body near the cancerous cells).

As well as being inconvenient for people who are already ill, if the diarrhoea is severe it can cause fluid and electrolyte losses, nutritional deficiencies and reduce quality of life. Perhaps more importantly though, the diarrhoea can often cause delays in the radiation treatment, or a reduction in the dose of radiation or even mean that the radiation treatment cannot continue at all, this means that the person will have a reduced chance of overcoming the cancer. Unfortunately, this side effect is common and most people who have radiotherapy to the abdomen, pelvis, or rectum will have diarrhoea. The diarrhoea which results from radiotherapy usually starts slowly a few days after the radiotherapy starts, gets worse as the treatment continues and stops a few weeks after the end of the course of treatment.

Probiotics are very effective for all the other types of diarrhoea that we have looked at, so can they help with this problem? Not as many studies have been undertaken as for some of the other causes of diarrhoea discussed above, but the results are promising. A review of this subject published in 2013 included 10 studies with 1,149 people taking part in all these studies. Five of the trials were of women with cervical or endometrial cancer who received pelvic radiotherapy, the others included both men and women who were having treatment for colorectal, bladder or prostatic cancer. The main finding was that probiotics reduced the incidence of diarrhoea by an average of 56%. The main probiotics used in these studies were Lactobacillus acidophilus, Bifidobacterium longum, Lactobacillus casei Shirota, Streptococcus thermophilus and various forms of Lactobacillus acidophilus.

In summary, we have seen that probiotics are an excellent way to both treat and prevent all of the most common types of diarrhoea, from infections, food poisoning or even radiation treatment.

Irritable bowel syndrome (IBS)

*** moderate amount of evidence of effectiveness

Now it's time to look at a condition that is not a form of diarrhoea, although this can certainly be a significant part of the disorder. Irritable Bowel Syndrome (IBS) is a common medical condition which affects the large bowel (AKA intestine or colon). The main symptoms are abdominal cramping, abdominal pain, bloating, gas, and, strangely, times of either diarrhoea or constipation. Unlike most of the types of diarrhoea discussed above, it is a chronic, long-term, condition. It is often confused with Inflammatory Bowel Disease (IBD), as the names of the conditions are similar. IBD will be discussed next, and, while not minimising the impact of IBS, IBD is a much more serious condition in terms of its effect on health.

Fortunately, few people with IBS have severe symptoms and often they can be managed reasonably well with dietary modifications, lifestyle changes and reducing stress levels. Others will need medication and counselling.

In Western countries, as many as one in five adults have signs and symptoms of IBS, although most do not seek medical help. Sufferers are usually less than 45 years old, twice as likely to be women and may well have other people in the family with the condition. It is a troublesome rather than a severe illness, but it is still important to see a doctor on a regular basis in order to make sure that there is nothing more serious going on. Symptoms that could potentially be signs of a more serious disease, such as bowel cancer, should be checked out. Such symptoms include: a persistent change in bowel habits; rectal bleeding; abdominal pain of increasing severity; or unexplained weight loss.

It is surprising, and disappointing, that for such a common and troublesome medical condition, little is known for sure about what causes it. People with IBS generally have contractions of the muscles that line the bowels that are stronger than in other people and also the part of the nervous system that lives in the GI tract can overreact and cause some of the symptoms.

As we do not know exactly what causes the condition, it is hard to predict if our friends the probiotics can help. One clue that they may be of use comes from studies that have found that people with IBS tend to have different intestinal microflora compared to people without IBS. Also, taking courses of antibiotics alters the bowel microflora and is linked to some cases of IBS. Some people have developed IBS suddenly after a GI tract infection, which would also alter their bowel microflora. So what does the research say? Again, we will look at one of the biggest reviews, the reason being that good reviews look at all the evidence and do not just pick out the positive research findings.

A review published in the *World Journal of Gastroenterology* included 20 trials which had enrolled over 1,400 people. The average duration of treatment with probiotics in the studies was only four weeks and as is usually the case, many different probiotic strains were used, mostly Lactobacillus and related species, with Lactobacillus rhamnosus GG and Bifidobacterium infantis being the ones that were looked at in more than one study. The review found that overall, use of probiotics led to a 23% chance of having an improvement in overall IBS symptoms. Mostly positive results were also seen in terms of specific symptoms including abdominal pain, bloating/distension, flatulence and overall quality of life.

Given that the condition is difficult to treat, this is quite an impressive result and the take-home message is that probiotics are well worth trying for people with IBS and they can continue taking them if they find that there is an improvement in their condition.

Inflammatory bowel disease

** small amount of evidence of effectiveness

As highlighted above, Inflammatory Bowel Disease (IBD) is a medical term describing conditions in which the intestine becomes inflamed (red and swollen). There are two major types of IBD: Crohn's disease and ulcerative colitis. Both of them are autoimmune diseases, in other words, the damage is actually caused by the body's own immune system attacking the intestines. There are a number of differences between the two conditions, the main ones being that Crohn's disease does not always affect the lower intestines, it causes patchy areas of inflammation, and the inflammation is often deep and causes narrowing and blockages. Ulcerative colitis on the other hand always affects the lower intestines, it causes continuous areas of inflammation, and the inflammation is often shallow and does not usually cause narrowing and blockages. While much rarer than IBS, as many as 1.4 million people in the USA and 2.2 million people in Europe suffer from these diseases.

The inflammation leads to similar symptoms in both diseases: abdominal pain, vomiting, diarrhoea, rectal bleeding, severe internal cramps and weight loss. A common complication which results from these symptoms is anaemia. Treatment is with medicines, some of which are potent inhibitors of the immune system and can have bad side effects. Sometimes, surgery of the bowel is required. It is common that there are periods of time when there is little or no disease activity and symptoms are minimal or even absent - a state that is called remission. Unfortunately, remission does not mean that the disease is cured and symptoms almost always come back after this period of respite.

The causes of IBD are not well understood and are thought to be due to complex interactions between environmental and genetic factors. Also, as with other conditions that we have already discussed and others we will discuss, the latest research suggests that alterations to intestinal bacteria can contribute to the development of IBD. People with the diseases have been found to have a 30-50 percent reduction in the number of different bacteria in their intestinal bioflora. Also, it has been discovered that people with IBD are more likely to have been prescribed antibiotics in the two to five year period before their diagnosis than people who do not have IBD.

Not surprisingly therefore, studies have looked at the effectiveness of probiotics for IBD. The Cochrane group have looked at all the relevant studies, and have compiled four reviews: looking at probiotics both for the induction of remission, and the maintenance of remission, for both Crohn's disease and ulcerative colitis.

Probiotics for *induction* of remission in ulcerative colitis

Four good quality studies were identified and included in the analysis, with a total of 244 people enrolled. In the studies all patients received standard treatment and some received probiotics as well. Unfortunately the conclusion was that people who had probiotics along with standard treatments had no additional benefit in terms of an induction of remission (i.e. starting a period of remission) or a reduction in symptoms compared to people who received standard treatments only.

Probiotics for *maintenance* of remission in ulcerative colitis

The aim of this review was to see if probiotics could help to keep people whose ulcerative colitis was in a state of remission in this state, i.e. do they help to stop the symptoms from coming back? Again, four good quality studies were identified and included in the analysis, with a larger total of 587 people enrolled. Three of the trials compared probiotics to the current "gold standard" of pharmaceutical medicines, mesalazine, and one trial compared probiotics with placebo; the studies ranged in duration from three to 12 months. There was no statistically significant difference between probiotics and mesalazine for the maintenance of remission in ulcerative colitis, with a relapse reported in 40% of patients in the probiotics group compared to 34% of patients in the mesalazine group (see previously for the definition of "statistically significant"). In the study where probiotics were compared with placebo, 75% of probiotic patients had relapsed after one year compared to 92% of placebo patients. Based on this relatively small amount of research, firm recommendations cannot be made. But this is promising, as probiotics were shown to be effective, in that they were better than placebo and even seemed to be nearly as effective as the current best pharmaceutical medicine.

Probiotics for *induction* of remission in Crohn's disease

Moving onto the less common Crohn's disease, and starting again with studies that have looked at whether probiotics could help to make the disease go into remission, the Cochrane review only found one good study of just 11 people. There did not appear to be a benefit in this study, but in reality, there is nowhere near enough evidence to comment and research is needed in this area.

Probiotics for *maintenance* of remission in Crohn's disease

Finally, when it comes to probiotics as a treatment to try to keep a person with Crohn's disease in a state of few symptoms, six small studies which enrolled 180 adults between them were included, and one study of 80 children. The probiotics used in the trials were Lactobacilli GG, Escherichia coli strain Nissle 1917, VSL#3 and Saccharomyces boulardii. Overall, none of the studies found a statistically significant benefit from probiotics. However, the trials were all very small, and in a number of them the probiotics appeared to be having a benefit. It is certainly possible that if larger trials were undertaken, then these benefits could be proven to be real. Therefore the study authors concluded that it is possible that larger studies might show that probiotics were in fact effective for this indication.

So, what can we conclude from all the research on probiotics for inflammatory bowel diseases? More research is needed, but there is some evidence that they may be effective, especially for maintenance of remission in people with ulcerative colitis.

Coeliac disease

* very little or no good evidence of effectiveness

As with Inflammatory Bowel Disease, Coeliac disease (also spelled as Celiac, also known as c(o)eliac sprue, nontropical sprue, endemic sprue, and gluten enteropathy) is an autoimmune disorder and in this condition the body's immune system attacks gliadin, a gluten protein that is found in wheat and other common grains including barley and rye. There is a strong genetic component and almost all people with the condition have one of two genes: HLA-DQ2 and DQ-8.

When an immune reaction to gliadin occurs, there is a cross-reaction with the small-bowel tissue, which becomes inflamed. This inflammation damages the villi which line the small intestine. Villi are small, finger-like projections that are crucial in terms of absorbing nutrients, as they effectively increase the surface area of this part of the GI tract, which is necessary for good absorption of nutrients from food. Therefore, in coeliac disease there is much reduced absorption of nutrients, which can cause anaemia and deficiencies of vitamins and minerals such as vitamin D, selenium, calcium and copper. The other symptoms are GI tract related, including pain and discomfort in the abdomen tract, chronic constipation and/or diarrhoea. People with coeliac disease also face an increased risk of intestinal cancer. There is only one known effective treatment and that is a lifelong gluten-free diet.

The prevalence of coeliac disease in adults in Western countries is around 1%, but it is often not diagnosed and people live with the symptoms for many years without realizing that they have the disease and that there is something they could be doing about it.

Not surprisingly, some researchers have looked at whether probiotics may be useful, but given that it is a relatively common condition, it is surprising that more research has not been undertaken. Studies have found that people with Coeliac disease have abnormalities in the intestinal microbiome, with reduced concentrations of Bifidobacterium species in particular. The potential usefulness of probiotics has also been demonstrated *in vitro* (i.e. in test tube studies) and in studies of animals.

Only a few studies have assessed probiotics as a treatment in humans. The best data has come from a small study of 22 adults which assessed the probiotic Bifidobacterium infantis natren life start strain super strain (Lifestart 2). Those who took the probiotic and not the placebo had a significant reduction in gastro-intestinal symptoms and blood tests showed that they had less inflammation.

So the take home message is to watch this space: more studies are needed and it is certainly possible that in the future we may find that probiotics are effective. But given their safety, as we discuss below, and low cost, they may be worth a try by people with Coeliac disease, who could continue taking them if they think that they help with their symptoms.

Helicobacter pylori infection

*** moderate amount of evidence of effectiveness

Before discussing in detail whether probiotics can help to treat a stomach infection caused by the bacteria Helicobacter pylori, it is well worth briefly telling the amazing story of the Australian doctor Barry Marshall, as not only is it very relevant to this section, it also illustrates how bacteria can be important for our health in ways we had not previously thought possible. In the 1980s around 10% of adults in Western countries suffered from stomach ulcers. As well as suffering from pain, many had severe bleeding from the ulcers, which could be fatal, and many had to have their stomach removed. This renegade doctor theorized that the bacteria Helicobacter pylori, which was present in very high levels in many patients with stomach ulcers and also stomach cancer, was often to blame and therefore antibiotics could be used to treat stomach ulcers. This was, at the time, a bizarre and outrageous suggestion, totally opposed to what mainstream medicine was saying, which was that the cause of the ulcers was usually stress. So he got some Helicobacter pylori bacteria from the stomach of a patient who was sick with stomach ulcers, stirred it into a broth, and drank it! After a few days, he developed gastritis, the precursor to an ulcer, and was very ill. Having demonstrated his theory effectively, he then bolstered it by taking antibiotics and curing himself. For this extraordinary work he was awarded a Nobel Prize in 1985. This story also demonstrates how new thinking can lead to better medical treatments, something that we are seeing right now with probiotics.

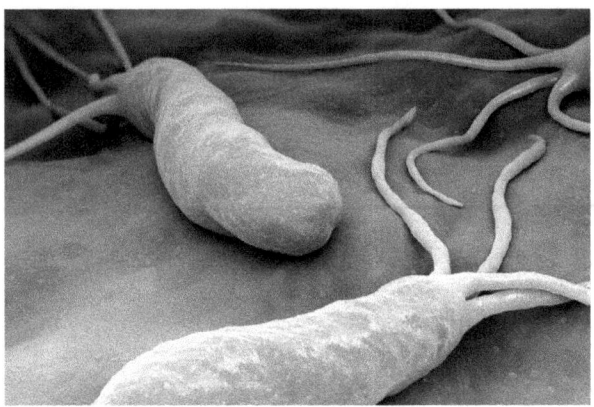

Helicobacter bacteria

About two-thirds of the world's population has Helicobacter pylori in their bodies but for most it does not cause ulcers or any other symptoms. For some people though, the bacteria attacks the lining of the stomach, which when intact, protects against the acid that the stomach makes to digest food. Damage from the bacteria means stomach acid can get through the lining causing problems such as gastritis and ulcers. Most treatments are based around antibiotics, for the reasons given above, medicines that reduce the production of stomach acid, medicines that protect the stomach wall lining, and often a combination of several medicines are used for the best results. However the commonly prescribed triple therapy of three medicines, the gold standard treatment for Helicobacter pylori eradication, is effective in only around 70% of patients, and so any new treatments would be welcome, especially given how common the condition is.

As I am sure you will have guessed, studies have looked at whether probiotics can help. There are several potential mechanisms by which probiotic supplements may help, including: modulating the immune system; reducing the side effects of medicines that are commonly used for this condition, enabling patients to continue taking them; and either killing, or at least stopping the growth of Helicobacter pylori.

Several studies have been undertaken, and a review published in 2013 looked at ten clinical trials which included nearly 1,500 patients. Although not conclusive, the researchers found that Lactobacillus-containing and Bifidobacterium-containing probiotics may have beneficial effects on the eradication of Helicobacter pylori infection and also appeared to reduce the side effects of other medications that were being taken to treat the condition.

So, 30 years later, we have a nice addition to Dr. Barry Marshall's story, with a different type of bacteria being ingested in order to help treat stomach ulcers.

Constipation

** small amount of evidence of effectiveness

This is clearly counterintuitive, given that most of this chapter has been discussing how useful probiotics are for many types of diarrhoea, but there is evidence that they may also be useful for exactly the opposite complaint, constipation.

Constipation is so common that almost everyone is affected at some time during his or her life, and at any given time, around 2% of the people in Western countries, particularly women and the elderly, are affected. The normal length of time between bowel movements ranges widely from person to person and a person is suffering from constipation when bowel movements become difficult or less frequent, compared to what is normal for that person. There is usually no underlying medical condition that is causing the problem and common causes include: inadequate fluid intake; inadequate fibre in the diet; a disruption of regular diet or routine, e.g. when traveling; inadequate activity or immobility; and stress. As well as a longer time between bowel movements, there can be associated symptoms including a sense of incomplete bowel movement, a swollen abdomen, abdominal pain or in severe cases, vomiting.

The best thing an affected person can do is to address and correct if necessary any of the lifestyle factors that may be causing or contributing to the problem, i.e. keep well hydrated, eat more fibre and do more exercise. Simple laxative medicines such as senna, lactulose, castor oil and Milk of Magnesia may help. The person can try several different ones, as there are a number of different ways in which they can work.

So in terms of treatments, can probiotics help? As with several of the conditions already discussed above, there is evidence demonstrating that there are differences in the intestinal microbiota between healthy people and people who suffer from chronic constipation. Another reason that they may work is that probiotics lower the pH in the colon, i.e. make it more acidic, by producing chemicals such as butyric acid, propionic acid, and lactic acid. We know that a lower pH increases movements of the colon and should, in theory at least, cause more bowel movements.

A review published in 2010 identified five good studies on this subject, but they were all quite small and the total number of people who took part was less than 400. Both children and adults took part in the studies, which compared probiotics to placebo. The probiotics assessed were Bifidobacterium lactis DN-173 010, E. coli Nissle 1917, Lactobacillus casei rhamnosus Lcr35, L. casei Shirota, and L. rhamnosus GG. The results were not conclusive and found that, overall, there appeared to be small benefits in terms of increasing the number of bowel movements, but the effect was quite small. In this situation, where some positive data is available but not enough to draw a firm conclusion or make a recommendation, which is a common situation for many medical products, particularly natural products, all we can say is that more research is needed and that a person can always try the treatment, and continue with it if it seems to be helping.

Chapter 5

NON GASTRO-INTESTINAL DISEASES

Until a decade or two ago, the idea that probiotics could have any effect outside of the GI tract was unheard of, and seemed to make no sense. Effects on the GI tract made sense, as that is where they travelled to and where they could have an effect. However, as we have seen above, the hundred trillion or so bacteria in our body play an important role in our immune system, and as our immune system protects us from many illnesses, and disorders of the immune system can cause many diseases. It is now understood that these bacteria can, and most definitely do, play an important role in a number of medical conditions outside of the GI tract.

For some of the conditions discussed below, not much research work has been done in humans at this stage, and so probiotics represent a potential treatment in the future. Therefore, the ratings given for probiotics for some of the conditions to follow will be quite low. However, we can be almost certain that research in the near future will prove that probiotics are effective for some of these conditions, and conditions that are not even discussed yet. Also, if you have one of these conditions but the current evidence for probiotics as a treatment is limited, then there is no harm in simply giving them a go and seeing if they benefit you. Although this book talks about the importance of clinical trials evidence, we are all different and for various reasons not everyone will benefit from a "proven" treatment, and some people certainly can benefit from a treatment that is "unproven".

RATING SYSTEM

* very little or no good evidence of effectiveness

** small amount of evidence of effectiveness

*** moderate amount of evidence of effectiveness

**** very good evidence of effectiveness

Immune system support

**** very good evidence of effectiveness

We will start with the big one, one of the main reasons that millions of people around the world take a probiotic capsule, or drink a probiotic drink every day, and that is because of the belief that they can help boost the immune system. On the surface this certainly makes sense, given that the micro-organisms in the body are a key part of the immune system and that probiotics, by definition, are beneficial micro-organisms. Millions of people clearly do believe that this is the case and take them daily, but it is controversial, and the UK NHS website states (wrongly in my view): *"...it's hard to see how swallowable bacteria could have an effect on conditions outside of the digestive tract."*

In some ways, whether probiotics can support or boost the immune system is quite a difficult question to answer. It may seem like a simple task, but in practice it is not easy to prove that probiotics do indeed bolster the immune system. There is not a simple blood test that we can do which gives us a measure of the immune system overall; if there was, we could simply do this test, give probiotics, and see if they improved the results of the test. In addition, there is still a huge amount that scientists do not know about the complexities and interconnections of the immune system, with new findings being published literally every day. However, researchers have looked at the effects of probiotics on different cells and chemicals of the immune system, and that is what we will cover in this section.

Another measure of whether the immune system has been boosted by probiotics could be to look at whether they stop people getting infections, as preventing and minimising the impact of infections is the primary role of the immune system. We have already seen how probiotics can help with GI tract infections, and the evidence for the use of probiotics for infections outside of the GI tract will be discussed in later parts of this chapter, where we will look at whether they can help reduce the incidence and/or help to treat, some specific, non-GI tract, infectious diseases. Finally, some diseases, such as the Inflammatory Bowel Diseases discussed previously, and other diseases discussed later, are a result of a malfunction of the immune system so that it harms the body or causes health issues (e.g. autoimmune diseases, allergies) and the effectiveness of probiotics for these conditions is also covered.

So you can see, it is not a simple task at all to answer the question of whether probiotics boost the immune system. In terms of effects on immune system cells and chemicals, it is, without being condescending to the reader, difficult to describe in simple terms, given the complexities of the immune system. *In vitro* (meaning research done in test tubes in laboratories) and *in-vivo* studies (those done in animals and humans) suggest that probiotics definitely do affect the immune response in positive ways. The following is a list of a number of beneficial effects on markers of the immune system that have been seen in the various studies:

EFFECTS OF PROBIOTICS ON SOME IMMUNE SYSTEM MARKERS

- Improving the body's own defence systems in several ways.
- Enhancement of the activity of natural killer cells.
- Modulation of non-specific host defences.
- Reversal of age-related decline in cytokine production.
- Induction of mucus production.
- Macrophage activation.
- Stimulation of secretory IgA.
- Stimulation of neutrophils.
- Inhibition of the release of inflammatory cytokines.
- Stimulation of elevated peripheral immunoglobulins.
- Modulation of dendritic cell surface phenotype and cytokine release.

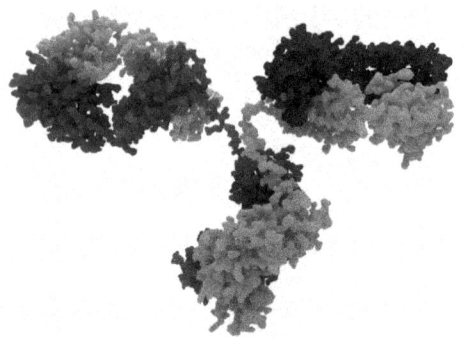

An antibody (aka immunoglobulin or Ig)

These are just some of the positive effects of probiotics on the immune system that have been found in studies in laboratories, in animals and in humans. However, the above improvements in markers of the immune system do not prove that there will be benefits to health on their own, they must be considered alongside studies looking at whether probiotics can help with infections and/or diseases caused by the immune system and as we have seen and will see, this is certainly the case.

Preventing upper respiratory tract infections

**** very good evidence of effectiveness

There are many different types of infections that we commonly get in our upper respiratory tracts. This part of the body starts at the nose and also includes the sinuses, tonsils, throat and larynx. (Pneumonia involves the lungs themselves and so is a lower respiratory tract infection and much more serious). Viruses cause most upper respiratory tract infections (URTIs), we are all very familiar with the most common of these, the common cold. The viruses that are usually responsible include rhinovirus, parainfluenza virus, coronavirus, adenovirus, respiratory syncytial virus, Coxsackie virus and influenza virus. Sore throats can be caused by bacteria as well as viruses, particularly one called Group A beta-haemolytic streptococcus.

Transmission of the micro-organisms which cause URTIs occurs by aerosol (e.g. sneezing), droplet, or direct hand-to-hand contact with infected secretions. Onset of symptoms occurs one to three days after exposure to the infectious agent, causing symptoms which include nasal congestion, sneezing, sore throat, cough and sometimes muscle aches.

Most URTIs occur more frequently during the cold winter months, partly because of more overcrowding in public areas. Adults develop an average of two to four colds per year, and children can experience up to 10 or 12 (the number we experience each year decreases as our immune system develops and we become immune to viruses and bacteria that we have previously encountered). The estimated economic impact of URTIs, excluding the more serious influenza, is estimated to be $40 billion a year in the USA alone. They are one of the main reasons why people visit their GP or pharmacist and one of the main reasons why people take time off school or work. Influenza epidemics occur every year in the winter and 40,000 to 60,000 people die each year as a result of influenza and its complications. Rest is recommended for people suffering from a URTI although there is no evidence that complete bed rest shortens the duration of illness.

So, can probiotics help? A Cochrane review published in 2015 addressed the issue of probiotics for preventing acute upper respiratory tract infections and included 13 clinical trials, which involved 3,720 children, adults and older people. The results were very positive indeed, with the reviews finding that probiotics:

- reduced the number of people experiencing any URTIs by around a half.
- reduced the number of people experiencing at least three episodes of URTI by around a half.
- reduced the average duration of a URTI by around two days.
- reduced the need to have an antibiotic prescription for a URTI by around two thirds.
- reduced the time off school for colds by around 90%.

These are quite remarkable results and, as we all get colds and other upper respiratory tract infections, it could well be argued that we are all likely to benefit from taking probiotics, particularly in the winter months, to reduce the number of colds and other URTIs we suffer from, and if we do get them, to likely reduce the time until we are back to normal.

Urogenital infections

A common reason that women take probiotics is to prevent and treat infections in the genital area; there are two main conditions that they are used for, both are discussed separately.

Bacterial vaginosis

**** very good evidence of effectiveness

This is a mild infection of the vagina caused by bacteria. As with the GI tract, there are normally a lot of "good" bacteria and some "bad" bacteria in the vagina, with the good ones helping to control the growth of the bad ones. In women with bacterial vaginosis this balance is altered such that there are too many bad bacteria and not enough good bacteria (especially Lactobacilli). Normally these lactobacilli produce a lot of acid, including lactic acid, and peroxide, these keep the pH of the vaginal low (i.e. acidic), which prevents the overgrowth of disease-causing bacteria. It is usually a mild problem that may well go away on its own after a few days. The most common symptom is an unpleasant smelling discharge, although around half of women who have bacterial vaginosis do not notice any symptom at all. It is usually not a serious condition, the exception being if it occurs in pregnancy, in which case it increases the risk of suffering a miscarriage and of having an infection of the uterus after the pregnancy. A doctor will often prescribe antibiotics for a week or so; metronidazole or clindamycin are the most common drugs, they are administered orally or intravaginally.

Given the main issue occurring in this condition, not enough good bacteria and too many bacteria, it would appear that this would be a condition that probiotics could help. The review of the studies found four suitable studies with around 400 women taking part in total. The studies were all quite different:

- in one study women took oral metronidazole and either probiotics or placebo, and a cure was achieved in 88% of women taking the additional probiotics compared to just 40% cured with the antibiotic alone.
- a study compared probiotic intravaginal capsules with intravaginal metronidazole gel, and 65% of the women using the probiotics were cured compared to just 33% of those using the antibiotic.
- in a study looking at the use of lactobacilli impregnated tampons, compared to normal tampons, there was no benefit from the probiotics.
- finally, a study compared vaginal tablets containing L. acidophilus and estriol (a hormone) to placebo tablets, with the cure rates being 88% and 14% respectively.

It was not possible to add up the results of these studies to give a single result (a "meta-analysis"), as the studies were all very different, but it is clear that probiotics are effective for this condition.

Vulvovaginal candidiasis

** small amount of evidence of effectiveness

Also known as Candidal vulvovaginitis, monilia or vaginal thrush, this is an infection of the vagina's mucous membranes by the fungus Candida albicans. About 20% of non-pregnant women aged 15 to 55 years have this fungus in the vagina and usually it is harmless and there are no symptoms. However, if there is overgrowth of the Candida albicans, then there can be a discharge, a burning sensation and/or an itchy rash in the affected area. Factors which can contribute to such an overgrowth include pregnancy, some oral contraceptive or hormone replacement therapy medications, antibiotics, diabetes, anaemia and an underperforming immune system. Around 75% of women will have this infection at some point in their lives.

As with bacterial vaginosis, a key factor in the development of candidal vulvovaginitis is an imbalance in the normal vaginal microflora, with a decrease in Lactobacilli bacteria and a subsequent overgrowth of Candida. Treatment is with antifungal creams, tablets or vaginal tablets. In around 5% of women it recurs repeatedly, and particularly in these cases, it is important to try to address any underlying medical problem which is making attacks more likely.

Probiotics are often taken to prevent and/or treat this condition. Some women have lots of yoghurt in their diets in order to get probiotics and some will put yoghurt in their vagina and report that it is effective. A 2006 review looked in detail at this topic. Firstly, the review noted that there were a number of good *in vitro* studies that have shown that Lactobacilli inhibit the growth of Candida albicans, and also inhibit adherence of the fungus to the vaginal wall. As for the more important clinical studies with women, unfortunately there were not many trials, and the ones that have occurred were quite small and not the best designed studies. That said, the evidence that is available generally concludes that Lactobacilli, especially Lactobacillus acidophilus, Lactobacillus rhamnosus GR-1 and Lactobacillus fermentum RC-14, do prevent the colonization and infection of the vagina by Candida albicans. These probiotics can be administered either orally or intravaginally. The review authors concluded, as I do, that although the evidence is weak, given the safety of probiotics, and low cost, they are well worth trying, particularly for women with frequent recurrence of the condition.

To finish this section on a more lighthearted note, it was interesting during the research for this section to see a probiotic product called Fermalac marketed for this condition. The product contains Lactobacilli which are referred to as *"the Xena warrior princesses of the vagina!"*

Ventilator-associated pneumonia

*** moderate amount of evidence of effectiveness

Another type of infection which doctors struggle to treat is called ventilator-associated pneumonia, shortened to VAP. Millions of people each year are admitted to intensive care units (ICUs). By definition they are already extremely unwell and they may be so ill that they need to be on a ventilator i.e. a machine that supports breathing. This procedure is only undertaken where absolutely necessary and is not without risks. A reasonably common problem that it can cause is that the lungs become infected i.e. it causes a pneumonia. It has been estimated that about half of all antibiotics given in the intensive care unit are for this reason. Around 20% of people who are ventilated will get pneumonia, those that get it usually need a longer time in ICU and in hospital, and around 10% of people will die from VAP.

Some doctors have tried administering probiotics to help prevent and treat this serious infection and in 2014 a Cochrane Review addressed the subject. Eight studies with nearly 1,100 patients were included in the review. As usual, Lactobacilli and Bifidobacterium species were the main probiotics tested. The main result was that the use of these probiotics reduced the chances of getting VAP by 30%. There was also some evidence, although it was weaker and not statistically significant, that they also reduce the number of deaths in ICU, the incidence of diarrhoea in patients on ventilators, the length of time spent in ICU, the length of time of the mechanical ventilation and the amount of antibiotics that were used.

So this, again, is very promising evidence. However, the level of evidence required before a treatment is incorporated into a hospital setting, especially one that involves the sickest of patients, is very high indeed, and more and bigger studies will have to be done to prove if probiotics are effective for preventing VAP. However, to me it illustrates just how far we have come in just a few decades, such that what was a fringe alternative medicine is not only used by millions of people around the world each day, but could soon be routinely given to some of the most ill people in the hospital.

Treating eczema

* very little or no good evidence of effectiveness

Eczema is also known as atopic dermatitis (meaning an inflammation of the skin due to allergy) and it's one of the three common childhood allergic diseases, the others being asthma and hayfever. Often, children who are prone to allergies will have eczema when they are babies, this goes away and then they have asthma when they are a bit older, and this goes away and they get hay fever when they are teenagers. There are many variations on this theme, but this so-called "allergic march" is often seen by family doctors who look after children from birth to adulthood.

Between 10–20 % of children have eczema at some stage, usually early in childhood, but many grow out of the condition and so fewer adults have it. The prevalence of these allergic diseases has increased over the last few decades and the possible reasons for this are discussed in the next section, as well as reasons as to why probiotics may be helpful.

In the short-term the main symptoms are itchy, red, dry skin. The symptom that people most often complain about is the itching (although babies cannot of course complain about this, they manifest it instead by scratching). There is often a vicious cycle of itching, followed by scratching, leading to skin damage which in turn leads to more itching.....this is called the "itch-scratch-itch" cycle. In the long-term, especially if treatments are not very effective, this can lead to skin scaling, thickening and discolouration. Although it can affect any part of the body, usually only certain areas of skin are affected, those areas being the creases of the elbows and knees, the face and the neck. There is a wide variation in the severity of the condition, ranging from a few small itchy areas for short periods of time, to almost the whole body being affected almost all the time. The latter state is very distressing for babies and their caregivers, and babies may be dressed in cotton clothes and have cotton gloves on to try to reduce the itching and scratching.

Standard medical treatments are emollients (moisturisers) and steroid creams and ointments, the former to try to stop the skin from being too dry, the latter to try to reduce the inflammation. If there are any known environmental factors which exacerbate the symptoms, such as soaps and detergents, pet fur, hot weather, or foods such as dairy products, then exposure to these should of course by reduced as much as is practical.

The intestinal microflora has been found to be different in people with eczema, in particular, there is a reduced proportion of Bifidobacteria species in the faeces of infants with eczema, which is one reason why some researchers think that changes in the intestinal microflora may cause or worsen eczema, and why probiotics may help.

12 studies which included nearly 800 participants were included in the analyses that were undertaken as part of a review of this subject. All the studies were undertaken in children, eight of the studies assessed the effect of probiotics on eczema in children who were less than 18 months old. All but one of the studies used a Lactobacillus species of probiotic as either the only probiotic, or one of a mixture. Overall, the results were disappointing, and there was no strong evidence that probiotics were better than placebo for reducing symptoms or severity. The authors stated that *"we conclude that probiotics are not an effective treatment for eczema."* It is possible that future studies, maybe with different probiotic strains or different doses may find an important effect, but at this stage, as opposed to preventing eczema as discussed next, probiotics are not an effective treatment for established eczema.

Preventing eczema and other allergic diseases

** small amount of evidence of effectiveness

There are various theories which try to explain the increasing prevalence of the allergies that we have seen over the last few decades. One of these hypotheses is the "linoleic acid hypothesis", which states that a possible explanation lies in the changing choice of dietary fats and the changes in the composition of the dietary fats in our food. Another hypothesis, the one that this author favours, is the "hygiene hypothesis". In layman's terms, this theory argues that we are much too clean these days, and have a much smaller exposure to dirt and micro-organisms than we did at the start of the century and prior to this time. For example, our families are much smaller (so there are fewer people coughing on us!), our food is more sterile, we are vaccinated against a number of infectious diseases, and if we do suffer from one, we often take antibiotics to treat the infection. All of this and more means than our immune systems do not have much to do and instead react against things in the environment (allergies) or even our own bodies (autoimmune diseases).

What allergies are we talking about? We have already mentioned eczema, asthma and hay fever above. Others include peanut allergy and other food allergies such as milk, soy, eggs, wheat, tree nuts, fish, and shellfish, and non-foods such as latex and some cleaning agents. Around 7% of children develop a food allergy.

A number of studies have looked at whether probiotics can prevent the development of these allergic conditions. As allergies almost always develop early in life, the studies have tended to look at the effects on infants. In some cases the probiotics were given to the infants themselves and in others they were given to the pregnant or breastfeeding mothers who pass them on. The studies tended to only include infants who were at high risk of developing allergic diseases, i.e. infants whose close family members had allergies, as this is the most important risk factor. The Cochrane Review on this subject included six studies which looked at the effects of probiotics on allergic diseases and/or food hypersensitivity and there were over 2,000 infants in these studies, meaning that we have a lot of good information. Overall, the results were disappointing: there was no good evidence that giving probiotics to infants, either directly or indirectly via the mother, reduced the chance of developing allergies in general, or more specifically food hypersensitivity, asthma or hayfever. The exception was eczema where the five studies that looked at this condition found an average of an 18% reduction in the chance of developing eczema.

Peanut allergy is an increasingly common problem and can be life-threatening. Probiotics may offer a hope with this condition after a study published in 2015 used the novel approach of using both probiotics and oral immunotherapy (OIT). OIT involves giving very small and increasing amounts of a substance that someone is allergic to, in order to increase their tolerance and even stop them being allergic at all. The probiotic Lactobacillus rhamnosus was used and in this study of 60 children this combination was effective: the children who received the combined OIT and probiotic treatment had a 20 times higher tolerance to peanuts than the placebo group. N.B. OIT should only be undertaken under the guidance of experienced medical professionals.

So overall, it is probably not worth giving infants probiotics for the purpose of reducing their chances of developing allergies. The exceptions are perhaps for peanut allergy and eczema, although more studies are needed. We have seen above that once eczema has developed then probiotics are unlikely to help, so if one or both parents have suffered from eczema, and want to reduce the chance of their children developing the condition, then probiotics can help to make this less likely.

Weight loss

** small amount of evidence of effectiveness

Early in 2014 the internet erupted with news that probiotics may help people to lose weight. Headlines included:

"Probiotics can help women with weight loss" - New York Daily News

"Yogurt Helps Women Lose Weight and Keep It Off" - Time

"Lose weight with probiotic bacteria" - Men's Health magazine

If true, then this would be a remarkable finding and also one with huge implications for public health. Obesity rates are rising rapidly around the world, particularly in children. Around one in 10 children are obese by the age of five in Western countries, and over a third are overweight or obese by the end of primary school. Health advocacy groups have called for a raft of measures to address the issue, including taxes on junk foods, and requirements for all schools to teach cooking and nutrition. The implications of being overweight are not just aesthetic: people who are overweight or obese have a much greater risk of developing a multitude of diseases from heart disease and Type 2 diabetes to bone and joint disease.

So was this media hype justified, and are probiotics an answer to this huge problem? The study which triggered all these headlines was published in the British Journal of Nutrition. The 125 overweight men and women in the study underwent a 12-week weight-loss diet, followed by a 12-week period aimed at maintaining body weight. Throughout the entire study, half the participants swallowed two pills daily containing probiotics from the Lactobacillus rhamnosus family, while the other half received a placebo. After the 12-week diet period, researchers observed an average weight loss of 4.4 kg in women in the probiotic group and 2.6 kg in the placebo group. Intriguingly, no differences in weight loss were observed among males in the two groups. After the 12-week maintenance period, the weight of the women in the placebo group had remained stable but the probiotic group had continued to lose weight, and the average was now 5.2 kg per person.

These are astonishing findings and so it is not surprising that so much interest was generated. As to how the probiotic supplement might work, a number of mechanisms have been suggested, including:

- In this study, the researchers also noted a drop in the appetite-regulating hormone leptin in those who took probiotics, and so maybe they reduce appetite?
- Other studies have found that the intestinal flora of obese individuals differs from that of thinner people.
- It has been suggested that this difference in the intestinal flora may be due to the fact that a diet high in fat and low in fibre promotes certain bacteria at the expense of others.
- Further, the hypothesis has been put forward that taking probiotics could help to reset the balance of the intestinal microbiota in favour of bacteria that promote a healthy weight.

Several other studies have also found that probiotics may help with weight loss. A study in the *European Journal of Clinical Nutrition* in 2011 found that people who drank fermented milk with a particular strain of Lactobacillus gasseri for 12 weeks had a reduction in abdominal fat and body weight. Another study published a year later found that people who consumed yoghurt containing two strains of probiotics experienced small losses in body fat, but no changes in body weight. There is also a lot of work that has been undertaken in animals that has found probiotics can reduce weight.

So what can we conclude? These are intriguing findings but it is a little early to strongly recommend probiotics for weight loss - we need more and bigger studies to confirm these findings first. There is also the strange and disappointing fact that they did not appear to help men at all. So I would not make a strong recommendation to take probiotics for weight loss, but it is certainly worth trying if this is an issue for you, and there are many other reasons to take probiotics, and weight loss may be a nice bonus!

Dental decay

** small amount of evidence of effectiveness

We have discussed the bacteria in the lower end of the GI tract earlier in the book and how probiotics can be effective for many diseases that occur there. But there is another part of the GI tract where the balance of bacteria is important and where too many harmful bacteria can cause a problem, and that is the mouth.

Dental caries (tooth decay) is a major oral health problem in most industrialised countries, affecting 60–90% of schoolchildren and the vast majority of adults. Globally, around 2.5 billion people, or 36%, have dental caries in their permanent teeth. Unlike some other medical conditions, this is very much a disease of Western countries, as we have much more sugar in our diets than in many developing countries.

The process by which it occurs starts with a small patch of softened (demineralised) enamel on the surface of a tooth, and then spreads into the softer, sensitive part of the tooth beneath the enamel (the dentin). The weakened enamel then collapses to form a cavity and the tooth is progressively destroyed. This destruction is caused by the action of acids on the enamel surface, and these acids are produced when sugars in foods and drinks react with bacteria present in a dental biofilm (plaque) which can be on the tooth surface. These acids cause demineralisation as they are responsible for a loss of calcium and phosphate from the enamel. So by understanding this mechanism we can see that there would be no tooth decay if the bacterial plaques were not present, and so the problem is very much a result of too many of the wrong type of bacteria.

Most of us have experienced the symptoms of pain, difficulty with eating, tooth loss, and in severe cases there can be abscess formation. The main prevention methods are all very familiar as well: regular cleaning of the teeth, a diet low in sugar and the contentious topic of adding small amounts of fluoride to the general water supply.

There are many types of bacteria in the mouth, but only a few specific species of bacteria are known to cause dental caries: Streptococcus mutans, Actinomyces spp. and Nocardia spp. are those that are most closely linked to dental caries.

A few studies have looked at probiotics as a method for reducing dental caries. A slight complication is that many probiotic products are delivered in yoghurt and other forms of dairy produce, and the high levels of calcium that they also deliver can also help to reduce demineralization of teeth. A review of the most important studies published in 2013 found that the effect of probiotics on the development of dental caries lesions was encouraging. 23 studies were analysed, around half of which looked at the effects in children and adolescents and the other half looked at the effects in adults. Most of the studies looked at whether probiotics could reduce levels of the main dental caries bacterium: Streptococcus mutans, and in most studies, a significant reduction was seen. Milk, yoghurt, powders, chewing gum and lozenges were amongst the methods used to deliver the probiotics, which were predominantly forms of Lactobacillus rhamnosus and Bifidobacterium lactis. In one intriguing study, ice-cream was used as the probiotic vehicle - the ice cream delivered a combination of Bifidobacterium lactis Bb-12 and Lactobacillus acidophilus La-5 to 40 adolescents and there were significant reductions in saliva levels of Streptococcus mutans.

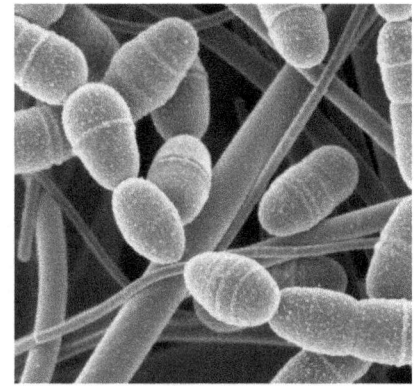

Streptococcus mutans

These results are promising, but studies have not yet shown that probiotics can actually stop tooth decay, they have simply shown that probiotics can reduce the levels of the main bacteria that are responsible. For this reason, probiotics cannot be strongly recommended for this reason alone, but as with weight loss above, an improvement in dental health may well be an additional benefit of a regular intake of probiotics.

Halitosis

*** moderate amount of evidence of effectiveness

As well as rotten teeth, another condition that can result from having too much of the wrong type of bacteria in the mouth, and further down the GI tract, is bad breath - formally known as halitosis. The causes of this embarrassing condition include eating foods with strong odours such as garlic or onion, which are eventually carried to the lungs and are present in breath, and poor mouth hygiene due to not cleaning your teeth regularly, which allows food particles to remain in the mouth and promote bacterial growth. It can also be caused by more serious diseases elsewhere in the body, such as respiratory tract infections (e.g. pneumonia, bronchitis, chronic sinus infections), diabetes, chronic acid reflux, and even liver or kidney problems.

Several small studies have looked at the potential effectiveness of probiotics and the results are promising:

- A series of studies used the anti-microbial chemical chlorhexidine to reduce the number of bacteria in the mouth, and then attempted to repopulate the tongue surface with the probiotic Streptococcus salivarius K12. The majority of study participants had reduced breath levels of volatile sulphur compounds, which cause much of the odour.
- Another small study used the probiotic Lactobacillus salivarius WB21 and xylitol in tablet form and found that oral malodour was significantly decreased after two weeks.
- Another small study with 25 participants tested a chewing gum with two strains of the probiotic Lactobacillus reuteri, and again, bad odours were reduced.
- A study using a strain of Escherichia coli found that it greatly improved bad breath that came from gastric gases.

- And finally, Japanese researchers gave subjects with halitosis low amounts of Lactobacillus salivarius and found that after a month, oral levels of sulphur-producing compounds had significantly decreased.

There have been several other smaller studies, and while probiotics have not been proven to be effective at this stage, as the studies are all quite small, if this is an issue for you then they are certainly worth trying, particularly the strains named in the summaries of the research above.

Cancer prevention

* very little or no good evidence of effectiveness

So we will finish our look at conditions which probiotics may help with by looking at one of the most important: cancer. However, it is important to emphasize that we are not talking here about probiotics being a *cure* for cancer. Some fringe alternative medicine advocates do claim this, but there is no good evidence at all to support this. Instead we will be looking at whether they may *prevent* people from getting cancer. Another role they certainly do have for some people with cancer, as discussed above, is in helping to reduce the symptoms of the disease and/or treatment and/or complications of the disease that people with cancer can experience. These include diarrhoea (including diarrhoea caused by radiation treatment) and constipation, which is a common side effect of some drugs which reduce pain.

We all know people who have had cancer, and here are some facts you may not know, courtesy of the World Health Organization:

- There are more than 100 types of cancers; any part of the body can be affected.
- In 2008, 7.6 million people died of cancer - 13% of all deaths worldwide.
- About 70% of all cancer deaths occur in low- and middle-income countries.
- Worldwide, the five most common types of cancer that kill men are (in order of frequency): lung, stomach, liver, colorectal and oesophagus.
- Worldwide, the five most common types of cancer that kill women

are (in the order of frequency): breast, lung, stomach, colorectal and cervical. In many developing countries, cervical cancer is the most common cancer.
- Tobacco use is the single largest preventable cause of cancer in the world causing 22% of cancer deaths.
- One fifth of all cancers worldwide are caused by a chronic infection, for example human papillomavirus (HPV) causes cervical cancer and hepatitis B virus (HBV) causes liver cancer.
- Cancers of major public health relevance such as breast, cervical and colorectal cancer can be cured if detected early and treated adequately.
- More than 30% of cancer could be prevented, mainly by not using tobacco, having a healthy diet, being physically active and moderating alcohol consumption. In developing countries up to 20% of cancer deaths could be prevented by immunization against the infection of HBV and HPV.

How could probiotics reduce the risk of getting cancer? Several theories and mechanisms have been suggested, including:

- It is thought that acidophilus probiotics in particular can neutralize cancer-causing agents (carcinogens) in the diet.
- Probiotics can certainly affect and "boost" the immune system and this more effective immune system may be better at destroying or inhibiting pre-cancerous cells in the body and stop them developing into cancer cells.

What does the research say? Currently, we do not have good clinical trials that show that probiotics can prevent cancer, but there is an increasing amount of laboratory, animal, and epidemiological data that, when combined, make a good case that this could be the case. Such research findings include:

- In vitro studies with LGG and Bifidobacteria have found that these probiotics reduce the levels of carcinogens in the GI tract.
- Milk that has been fermented by L. acidophilus has been shown to slow or prevent the growth of breast and colon cancer cells grown in the laboratory.
- Animals that are given L. acidophilus are less prone to DNA damage

in the colon after being given known carcinogens, suggesting acidophilus might have a preventative effect on colon cancer.

So to conclude, we do not currently have proof that probiotics can prevent cancer, and they cannot be recommended for this reason. But there are lots of good reasons to take probiotics and an added bonus might be a reduced chance of developing cancer, particularly cancer of the colon.

Chapter 6
SAFETY

So we will finish our look at probiotics by discussing an aspect that often gets forgotten: safety. For any health product that you might consider taking, as well as the cost, it is important to take into account the balance between the likely health improvements and the possible side effects, i.e. between benefits and risks. So far we have seen that there are lots of potential benefits from taking probiotics, and in fact they are proven to be effective in terms of preventing and/or treating a number of common and important medical conditions. There is a strong case that most people would benefit from taking them each day in order to have a stronger immune system, suffer from fewer infections and more speculatively, maybe even lose weight or reduce the chances of developing cancer.

There is a widely held but false belief amongst many supporters of natural health products that natural products are inherently safe, as opposed to synthetic chemicals, but this is simply not true. In fact, anything that you ingest has the potential to harm you. Usually, the risk of harm is related to the amount (i.e. dose) of what is ingested, for example, drinking gallons of water in a day can actually be fatal. There are dozens of examples of how natural products that may on the surface appear to be totally safe may not be and a good example is amygdalin. It is extracted from apricot and almond kernels and is a popular alternative medicine amongst people with cancer. However, under certain conditions amygdalin breaks down into glucose, benzaldehyde, and most importantly, hydrogen cyanide, the latter being extremely poisonous.

So what are the possible mechanisms by which probiotics might cause harm? There are two main areas of potential concern. Firstly, by administering live micro-organisms, could these micro-organisms actually cause diseases? And secondly, can probiotics cause damage to the GI tract, rather than protecting it?

To answer the first question, one of the diseases that probiotics could in theory cause is endocarditis, an infection of the inner lining of the heart. This is an uncommon but serious condition which can be fatal and in some cases the bacteria responsible have been found to be lactic acid bacteria, which are of course one of the commonest species of probiotic. Another form of infection which probiotic micro-organisms could also potentially cause is sepsis, which is a potentially life-threatening condition triggered by an infection whereby the body's immune system goes into overdrive, setting off a series of reactions including widespread inflammation, swelling and blood clotting.

Should we be concerned that probiotics may cause serious infections? In a word, no - safety data from studies, and other information gathered from case reports is very reassuring. There are very few cases of endocarditis, or sepsis, or any other infection that have been suspected to have been caused by probiotics. Also, in almost all of the few cases where probiotics were suspected to be responsible, there are exceptional circumstances and usually the person has been extremely unwell and/or their immune system has not been fully functional, as can occur, for example, in people with HIV infection or people who have had a bone marrow transplant.

As for the second area of concern, whether probiotics can cause GI tract toxicity, again the data available is very reassuring. There are a few theoretical ways that probiotics could harm the GI tract, for example by producing harmful chemicals, but there are only a few case studies which have suggested that this may have occurred, and otherwise little justification for these concerns based on the published medical literature.

If there were any substantial health concerns, then it is likely that people with more serious illnesses whose health is already compromised would be most likely to suffer harm, so it is useful to look at the safety of probiotics in such people and a review has done just that. A 2013 review looked at the safety of probiotics in people with cancer. 17 studies with over 1,500 participants were included in this review, and there were only five case reports of probiotic-related bacteraemia. In other words, for around 99.7% of people with cancer, probiotics are safe and the safety profile will be much higher still in people without serious illnesses, which is the vast majority of people who take a regular dose of probiotics.

A bigger review has been undertaken by The Agency for Healthcare Research and Quality. They particularly focussed on six of the commonest probiotics that are used; Lactobacillus, Bifidobacterium, Saccharomyces, Streptococcus, Enterococcus and Bacillus. The report concluded that there was no strong evidence that people using probiotic organisms experienced more GI side effects, or infections, compared to participants in control groups of the studies.

So overall, probiotics are remarkably safe. Care should be taken in high-risk people, e.g. those with HIV / AIDS or who are critically ill. Also, preparations containing Lactobacillus species preparations are not advised for people with a hypersensitivity to lactose or milk and those containing Saccharomyces boulardii are not advised for people with a yeast allergy. Clinical data is limited, but there are no reports of harmful results associated with the use of probiotics in late-term pregnancies or in those who are breast-feeding. The vast majority of people will have no problems though. Around 20 billion doses of probiotics are taken every year.....**So are you going to take probiotics?**

Appendix
FURTHER READING

CHAPTER 1

Sanders, Mary Ellen. "Probiotics: definition, sources, selection, and uses." Clinical infectious diseases 46.Supplement 2 (2008): S58-S61.

Fuller, Roy. "History and development of probiotics." Probiotics. Springer Netherlands, 1992. 1-8.

Schrezenmeir, Jürgen, and Michael de Vrese. "Probiotics, prebiotics, and synbiotics—approaching a definition." The American journal of clinical nutrition 73.2 (2001): 361s-364s.

Salminen, S., et al. "Probiotics: how should they be defined?." Trends in food science & technology 10.3 (1999): 107-110.

Reid, Gregor, et al. "Potential uses of probiotics in clinical practice." Clinical microbiology reviews 16.4 (2003): 658-672.

Lee, Yuan-Kun, and Seppo Salminen. "The coming of age of probiotics." Trends in Food Science & Technology 6.7 (1995): 241-245.

Gomes, Ana MP, and F. Xavier Malcata. "Bifidobacterium spp. and Lactobacillus acidophilus: biological, biochemical, technological and therapeutic properties relevant for use as probiotics." Trends in Food Science & Technology 10.4 (1999): 139-157.

de Vrese, Michael, and J. Schrezenmeir. "Probiotics, prebiotics, and synbiotics." Food biotechnology. Springer Berlin Heidelberg, 2008. 1-66.

Holzapfel, Wilhelm H., and Ulrich Schillinger. "Introduction to pre-and probiotics." Food Research International 35.2 (2002): 109-116.

Ziemer, Cherie J., and Glenn R. Gibson. "An overview of probiotics, prebiotics and synbiotics in the functional food concept: perspectives and future strategies." International Dairy Journal 8.5 (1998): 473-479.

Fooks, Laura J., Roy Fuller, and Glenn R. Gibson. "Prebiotics, probiotics and human gut microbiology." International dairy journal 9.1 (1999): 53-61.

Shah, Nagendra P. "Functional foods from probiotics and prebiotics." Food technology 55.11 (2001): 46-46.

Tuohy, Kieran M., et al. "Using probiotics and prebiotics to improve gut health." Drug discovery today 8.15 (2003): 692-700.

CHAPTER 2

Saxelin, Maija. "Probiotic formulations and applications, the current probiotics market, and changes in the marketplace: a European perspective." Clinical infectious diseases 46.Supplement 2 (2008): S76-S79.

Young, John. "European market developments in prebiotic-and probiotic-containing foodstuffs." The British journal of nutrition 80.4 (1998): S231-3.

Foligné, Benoit, Catherine Daniel, and Bruno Pot. "Probiotics from research to market: the possibilities, risks and challenges." Current opinion in microbiology 16.3 (2013): 284-292.

Champagne, Claude P., et al. "Recommendations for the viability assessment of probiotics as concentrated cultures and in food matrices." International journal of food microbiology 149.3 (2011): 185-193.

Siro, Istvan, et al. "Functional food. Product development, marketing and consumer acceptance—A review." Appetite 51.3 (2008): 456-467.

Senok, A. C., A. Y. Ismaeel, and G. A. Botta. "Probiotics: facts and myths." Clinical Microbiology and Infection 11.12 (2005): 958-966.

Sanders, Mary Ellen, and Jos Huis. "Bringing a probiotic-containing functional food to the market: microbiological, product, regulatory and labeling issues." Lactic Acid Bacteria: Genetics, Metabolism and Applications. Springer Netherlands, 1999. 293-315.

Scarpellini, E. M. I. D. I. O., et al. "Probiotics: which and when?." Digestive diseases (Basel, Switzerland) 26.2 (2007): 175-182.

Salminen, Seppo, et al. "Lactic acid bacteria in health and disease." Lactic acid bacteria. (1993): 199-225.

Ljungh, A., and T. Wadstrom. "Lactic acid bacteria as probiotics." Current issues in intestinal microbiology 7.2 (2006): 73-90.

Bezkorovainy, Anatoly. "Probiotics: determinants of survival and growth in the gut." The American journal of clinical nutrition 73.2 (2001): 399s-405s.

Krasaekoopt, Wunwisa, Bhesh Bhandari, and Hilton Deeth. "Evaluation of encapsulation techniques of probiotics for yoghurt." International Dairy Journal 13.1 (2003): 3-13.

CHAPTER 3

Ouwehand, Arthur C., et al. "Probiotics: mechanisms and established effects." International Dairy Journal 9.1 (1999): 43-52.

Saulnier, Delphine M., Sofia Kolida, and Glenn R. Gibson. "Microbiology of the human intestinal tract and approaches for its dietary modulation." Current pharmaceutical design 15.13 (2009): 1403-1414.

Vitetta, Luis, et al. "A review of the pharmacobiotic regulation of gastro-intestinal inflammation by probiotics, commensal bacteria and prebiotics." Inflammopharmacology 20.5 (2012): 251-266.

Boirivant, Monica, and Warren Strober. "The mechanism of action of probiotics." Current opinion in gastroenterology 23.6 (2007): 679-692.

Vanderpool, Charles, Fang Yan, and D. Brent Polk. "Mechanisms of probiotic action: implications for therapeutic applications in inflammatory bowel diseases." Inflammatory bowel diseases 14.11 (2008): 1585-1596.

Sherman, Philip M., Juan C. Ossa, and Kathene Johnson-Henry. "Unraveling mechanisms of action of probiotics." Nutrition in Clinical Practice 24.1 (2009): 10-14.

Collado, M. Carmen, et al. "Protection mechanism of probiotic combination against human pathogens: in vitro adhesion to human intestinal mucus." Asia Pacific journal of clinical nutrition 15.4 (2006): 570-575.

Hemaiswarya, S., et al. "Mechanism of action of probiotics." Brazilian Archives of Biology and Technology 56.1 (2013): 113-119.

Corr, Sinead C., Colin Hill, and Cormac GM Gahan. "Understanding the mechanisms by which probiotics inhibit gastro-intestinal pathogens." Advances in food and nutrition research 56 (2009): 1-15.

Mack, David R., and Sylvie Lebel. "Role of probiotics in the modulation of intestinal infections and inflammation." Current opinion in gastroenterology 20.1 (2004): 22-26.

CHAPTER 4

D'Souza, Aloysius L., et al. "Probiotics in prevention of antibiotic associated diarrhoea: meta-analysis." Bmj 324.7350 (2002): 1361.

Allen, Stephen J., et al. "Probiotics for treating infectious diarrhoea." The Cochrane Library (2003).

Sazawal, Sunil, et al. "Efficacy of probiotics in prevention of acute diarrhoea: a meta-analysis of masked, randomised, placebo-controlled trials." The Lancet infectious diseases 6.6 (2006): 374-382.

Canani, Roberto Berni, et al. "Probiotics for treatment of acute diarrhoea in children: randomised clinical trial of five different preparations." Bmj 335.7615 (2007): 340.

Surawicz, Christina M. "Probiotics, antibiotic-associated diarrhoea and Clostridium difficile diarrhoea in humans." Best Practice & Research Clinical Gastroenterology 17.5 (2003): 775-783.

Isolauri, E. "Probiotics for infectious diarrhoea." Gut 52.3 (2003): 436-437.

Parkes, Gareth C., Jeremy D. Sanderson, and Kevin Whelan. "The mechanisms and efficacy of probiotics in the prevention of Clostridium difficile-associated diarrhoea." The Lancet infectious diseases 9.4 (2009): 237-244.

Videlock, E. J., and F. Cremonini. "Meta-analysis: probiotics in antibiotic-associated diarrhoea." Alimentary pharmacology & therapeutics 35.12 (2012): 1355-1369.

Hempel, Susanne, et al. "Probiotics for the prevention and treatment of antibiotic-associated diarrhea: a systematic review and meta-analysis." JAMA 307.18 (2012): 1959-1969.

Johnston, Brad C., et al. "Probiotics for the prevention of pediatric antibiotic-associated diarrhea." The Cochrane Library (2007).

McFarland, Lynne V. "Meta-analysis of probiotics for the prevention of traveler's diarrhea." Travel Medicine and Infectious Disease 5.2 (2007): 97-105.

Delia, P., et al. "Use of probiotics for prevention of radiation-induced diarrhea." World journal of gastroenterology: WJG 13.6 (2007): 912-915.

Moayyedi, Paul, et al. "The efficacy of probiotics in the treatment of irritable bowel syndrome: a systematic review." Gut 59.3 (2010): 325-332.

Whorwell, Peter J., et al. "Efficacy of an encapsulated probiotic Bifidobacterium infantis 35624 in women with irritable bowel syndrome." The American journal of gastroenterology 101.7 (2006): 1581-1590.

Hedin, Charlotte, Kevin Whelan, and James O. Lindsay. "Evidence for the use of probiotics and prebiotics in inflammatory bowel disease: a review of clinical trials." Proceedings of the Nutrition Society 66.03 (2007): 307-315.

Rolfe, Vivien E., et al. "Probiotics for maintenance of remission in Crohn's disease." The Cochrane Library (2006).

Butterworth, Andrew D., Adrian G. Thomas, and Anthony Kwaku Akobeng. "Probiotics for induction of remission in Crohn's disease." The Cochrane Library (2008).

Mallon, Peter T., et al. "Probiotics for induction of remission in ulcerative colitis." The Cochrane Library (2007).

Naidoo, Khimara, et al. "Probiotics for maintenance of remission in ulcerative colitis." The Cochrane Library (2011).

Collado, Maria Carmen, et al. "Specific duodenal and faecal bacterial groups associated with paediatric coeliac disease." Journal of clinical pathology 62.3 (2009): 264-269.

Smecuol, Edgardo, et al. "Exploratory, randomized, double-blind, placebo-controlled study on the effects of Bifidobacterium infantis natren life start strain super strain in active celiac disease." Journal of clinical gastroenterology 47.2 (2013): 139-147.

Tong, J. L., et al. "Meta-analysis: the effect of supplementation with probiotics on eradication rates and adverse events during Helicobacter pylori eradication therapy." Alimentary pharmacology & therapeutics 25.2 (2007): 155-168.

Wang, Zhen-Hua, Qin-Yan Gao, and Jing-Yuan Fang. "Meta-analysis of the efficacy and safety of Lactobacillus-containing and Bifidobacterium-containing probiotic compound preparation in Helicobacter pylori eradication therapy." Journal of clinical gastroenterology 47.1 (2013): 25-32.

Chmielewska, Anna, and Hania Szajewska. "Systematic review of randomised controlled trials: probiotics for functional constipation." World journal of gastroenterology: WJG 16.1 (2010): 69.

Banaszkiewicz, Aleksandra, and Hania Szajewska. "Ineffectiveness of Lactobacillus GG as an adjunct to lactulose for the treatment of constipation in children: a double-blind, placebo-controlled randomized trial." The Journal of pediatrics 146.3 (2005): 364-369.

CHAPTER 5

Perdigon, G., et al. "Immune system stimulation by probiotics." Journal of dairy science 78.7 (1995): 1597-1606.

Galdeano, C. Maldonado, and G. Perdigon. "The probiotic bacterium Lactobacillus casei induces activation of the gut mucosal immune system through innate immunity." Clinical and Vaccine Immunology 13.2 (2006): 219-226.

McCracken, V. J., H. R. Gaskins, and G. W. Tannock. "Probiotics and the immune system." Probiotics: a critical review. (1999): 85-111.

Perdigon, G., et al. "Study of the possible mechanisms involved in the mucosal immune system activation by lactic acid bacteria." Journal of Dairy Science 82.6 (1999): 1108-1114.

Hao, Qiukui, et al. "Probiotics for preventing acute upper respiratory tract infections." The Cochrane Library (2011).

Maldonado, José, et al. "Human milk probiotic Lactobacillus fermentum CECT5716 reduces the incidence of gastro-intestinal and upper respiratory tract infections in infants." Journal of pediatric gastroenterology and nutrition 54.1 (2012): 55-61.

Hatakka, Katja, et al. "Effect of long term consumption of probiotic milk on infections in children attending day care centres: double blind, randomised trial." Bmj 322.7298 (2001): 1327.

Abad, C. L., and N. Safdar. "The role of lactobacillus probiotics in the treatment or prevention of urogenital infections—a systematic review." Journal of Chemotherapy 21.3 (2009): 243-252.

Senok, Abiola C., et al. "Probiotics for the treatment of bacterial vaginosis." The Cochrane Library (2009).

Andreu, Antonia. "Lactobacillus as a probiotic for preventing urogenital infections." Reviews in Medical Microbiology 15.1 (2004): 1-6.

Falagas, Matthew E., Gregoria I. Betsi, and Stavros Athanasiou. "Probiotics for prevention of recurrent vulvovaginal candidiasis: a review." Journal of Antimicrobial Chemotherapy 58.2 (2006): 266-272.

Siempos, Ilias I., Theodora K. Ntaidou, and Matthew E. Falagas. "Impact of the administration of probiotics on the incidence of ventilator-associated pneumonia: A meta-analysis of randomized controlled trials*." Critical care medicine 38.3 (2010): 954-962.

Morrow, Lee E., Marin H. Kollef, and Thomas B. Casale. "Probiotic prophylaxis of ventilator-associated pneumonia: a blinded, randomized, controlled trial." American journal of respiratory and critical care medicine 182.8 (2010): 1058-1064.

Boyle, R. J., et al. "Probiotics for the treatment of eczema: a systematic review." Clinical & Experimental Allergy 39.8 (2009): 1117-1127.

Boyle, Robert John, et al. "Probiotics for treating eczema." The Cochrane Library (2008).

Wickens, Kristin, et al. "A differential effect of 2 probiotics in the prevention of eczema and atopy: a double-blind, randomized, placebo-controlled trial." Journal of Allergy and Clinical Immunology 122.4 (2008): 788-794.

Ouwehand, Arthur C. "Antiallergic effects of probiotics." The Journal of nutrition 137.3 (2007): 794S-797S.

Kalliomäki, Marko, et al. "Probiotics in primary prevention of atopic disease: a randomised placebo-controlled trial." The Lancet 357.9262 (2001): 1076-1079.

Rautava, Samuli, Marko Kalliomäki, and Erika Isolauri. "Probiotics during pregnancy and breast-feeding might confer immunomodulatory protection against atopic disease in the infant." Journal of allergy and clinical immunology 109.1 (2002): 119-121.

Nurmatov, Ulugbek, et al. "Allergen-specific oral immunotherapy for peanut allergy." The Cochrane Library (2012).

Santacruz, Arlette, et al. "Interplay between weight loss and gut microbiota composition in overweight adolescents." Obesity 17.10 (2009): 1906-1915.

Delzenne, Nathalie M., et al. "Targeting gut microbiota in obesity: effects of prebiotics and probiotics." Nature Reviews Endocrinology 7.11 (2011): 639-646.

Sweeney, Timothy E., and John M. Morton. "The human gut microbiome: a review of the effect of obesity and surgically induced weight loss." JAMA surgery 148.6 (2013): 563-569.

Näse, Leena, et al. "Effect of long-term consumption of a probiotic bacterium, Lactobacillus rhamnosus GG, in milk on dental caries and caries risk in children." Caries research 35 (2001): 412-20.

Stecksén-Blicks, C., I. Sjöström, and S. Twetman. "Effect of long-term consumption of milk supplemented with probiotic lactobacilli and fluoride on dental caries and general health in preschool children: a cluster-randomized study." Caries research 43.5 (2008): 374-381.

Anderson, M. H., and W. Shi. "A probiotic approach to caries management." Pediatric dentistry 28.2 (2006): 151-153.

Iwamoto, Tomoyuki, et al. "Effects of probiotic Lactobacillus salivarius WB21 on halitosis and oral health: an open-label pilot trial." Oral Surgery, Oral Medicine, Oral Pathology, Oral Radiology, and Endodontology 110.2 (2010): 201-208.

Burton, J. P., C. N. Chilcott, and J. R. Tagg. "The rationale and potential for the reduction of oral malodour using Streptococcus salivarius probiotics." Oral Diseases 11.s1 (2005): 29-31.

Wollowski, Ingrid, Gerhard Rechkemmer, and Beatrice L. Pool-Zobel. "Protective role of probiotics and prebiotics in colon cancer." The American journal of clinical nutrition 73.2 (2001): 451s-455s.

Rafter, Joseph. "Probiotics and colon cancer." Best Practice & Research Clinical Gastroenterology 17.5 (2003): 849-859.

Liong, Min-Tze. "Roles of probiotics and prebiotics in colon cancer prevention: Postulated mechanisms and in-vivo evidence." International journal of molecular sciences 9.5 (2008): 854-863.

CHAPTER 6

Didari, Tina, et al. "A systematic review of the safety of probiotics." Expert opinion on drug safety 13.2 (2014): 227-239.

Shanahan, Fergus. "A commentary on the safety of probiotics." Gastroenterology Clinics of North America 41.4 (2012): 869-876.

Hempel, Susanne, et al. "Safety of probiotics to reduce risk and prevent or treat disease." (2011).

Redman, M. G., E. J. Ward, and R. S. Phillips. "The efficacy and safety of probiotics in people with cancer: a systematic review." Annals of Oncology (2014): mdu106.

AlFaleh, K., and J. Anabrees. "Efficacy and safety of probiotics in preterm infants." Journal of neonatal-perinatal medicine 6.1 (2013): 1-9.

Gupta, R. "Lack of demonstrated safety and efficacy of probiotics in HIV patients." HIV medicine 14.8 (2013): 516-516.

Wang, Zhen-Hua, Qin-Yan Gao, and Jing-Yuan Fang. "Meta-analysis of the efficacy and safety of Lactobacillus-containing and Bifidobacterium-containing probiotic compound preparation in Helicobacter pylori eradication therapy." Journal of clinical gastroenterology 47.1 (2013): 25-32.

Morrow, Lee E., Vijaya Gogineni, and Mark A. Malesker. "Synbiotics and probiotics in the critically ill after the PROPATRIA trial." Current Opinion in Clinical Nutrition & Metabolic Care 15.2 (2012): 147-150.

www.ingramcontent.com/pod-product-compliance
Lightning Source LLC
Chambersburg PA
CBHW071120030426
42336CB00013BA/2153